You Can Do This!

Surviving Breast Cancer without Losing Your Sanity or Your Style

~~~~~~~~~~~~~

ELISHA DANIELS AND KELLEY TUTHILL,
WITH ANN PARTRIDGE, M.D., M.P.H.

**Andrews McMeel
Publishing, LLC**
Kansas City • Sydney • London

ISBN-13: 978-0-7407-8575-7
ISBN-10: 0-7407-8575-3

Library of Congress Control Number: 2009929575

10 11 12 13 MLT 10 9 8 7 6 5 4 3 2

This book is intended as a reference volume only, not a medical manual. Decisions about the need for or the type of medical treatment for any particular illness or problem should only be made after consultation with your doctor and family. This book is designed to give you information to assist you in making those decisions with the help of your doctor. It is not intended as a substitute for any treatment that may have been prescribed by your doctor. Mention of specific companies, organizations, or authorities in this book does not imply endorsement by the publisher, nor does mention of specific companies, organizations, or authorities imply that they endorse this book.

www.andrewsmcmeel.com

ATTENTION: SCHOOLS AND BUSINESSES
Andrews McMeel books are available at quantity discounts with bulk purchase for educational, business, or sales promotional use. For information, please write to: Special Sales Department, Andrews McMeel Publishing, LLC, 1130 Walnut Street, Kansas City, Missouri 64106.

CONTENTS

by Evelyn H. Lauder

In the collective fight against breast cancer, it is important to reflect on the individual women who lead this battle daily. These women have inspired and continue to inspire my work in the world of breast cancer research. In October 1992, I launched a project with the Estée Lauder Companies to mark National Breast Cancer Awareness Month. Estée Lauder counters across the country began distributing pink ribbons and breast self-exam instruction cards (over 85 million have now been distributed). The message was out and I was just beginning. I made an important decision to dedicate myself to improving treatment and finding a cure for this all-too-common disease.

From the outset, I knew that funding for lifesaving breast cancer research was at an unspeakably low level. My plan was to raise as much money as possible for the all-important work of breast cancer scientists. At the time (1993), no other organization was focused solely on coordinated translational research. With this in mind, I founded The Breast Cancer Research Foundation (BCRF), which has the single-purpose mission of seeking out the most creative and promising clinical and translational ideas, and providing funds to accelerate their progress. BCRF is about fueling the scientific discoveries that are changing the futures of women everywhere.

In the last sixteen years, we have seen remarkable strides in treatment thanks to our scientific advisory board and committee headed by Dr. Larry Norton and Dr. Clifford Hudis from Memorial Sloan-Kettering Cancer Center. Early detection, quality-of-life care, and potential prevention of breast cancer are topics of study as well. Science is an art form and funding is transformative. Time and time again, we hear from the brightest investigators that BCRF's funding has allowed for creativity, collaboration, and progress. We must provide able minds with resources to carry out their critical research work. BCRF's efforts are far from over. I always say that we aim for the day that we put ourselves out of business. I know that day will come with adequate funding.

Through BCRF, I have met incredibly strong women with some very important lessons to share. They are survivors in every sense of the word. While doctors and researchers wage their own war on cancer, I know there are 2 million women like Elisha Daniels and Kelley Tuthill facing an unthinkable diagnosis and every difficult decision that ensues. I so admire their ability to pick themselves up, often with no hair and weak bodies, and move forward on sheer spunk and determination.

Elisha and Kelley have a great message for us all: Cancer does not diminish a woman's beauty. I have witnessed women emerge from cancer more beautiful, more informed, and much stronger. I love the practical advice this book puts forth: Surround yourself with people you love; remain in control of your own care; and look good to feel good. Cancer can be met with sanity and style.

When I established BCRF, my goal was to create an organization to sponsor the very best breast cancer research in an effort to achieve prevention and a cure. This is my way of supporting each woman with breast cancer and celebrating each survivor. For women like Elisha and Kelley, I vow to continue BCRF's work until we eliminate this disease once and for all.

My utmost thanks goes to both of them for their loyal support, and for sharing their personal experiences and guidance to help others through this challenging experience. Elisha and Kelley will make the journey much more manageable for any woman and her closest loved ones who read this book. They speak intimately to the reader with tremendous understanding and compassion.

"You are going to get through this. I can't promise you that, but you have to believe it."

That's what a very smart doctor said to Kelley when she was diagnosed with breast cancer. That doctor's name is Hope, so Kelley took that as a good omen and listened to her. Having hope is a pretty good place to start after being given a diagnosis as devastating as cancer. For many of us, treatment will last at least a year and bring some of the biggest physical challenges we've ever faced. But it's the mental strength and positive attitude that will carry you. Oh, and if you're lucky, the love and support of those around you.

Kelley was thirty-six years old when she discovered a lump shortly after giving birth to her second daughter. Her husband, Brendan, urged her to get it checked out, and she went to her doctor. Kelley is so grateful that the doctor sent her for more testing even though they both thought it would be nothing. A mammogram and ultrasound confirmed the lump was cancer. It was a few days before Christmas 2006, and Kelley's children were just two and six months old. She had no family history of the disease and had never had a mammogram before because of her age. Further testing showed the cancer had spread to the lymph nodes and would require a mastectomy, chemotherapy, and radiation, and hormone therapy. Kelley, a television news reporter, worked as much as possible throughout treatment and documented her journey in a video and written diary that you can find at http://www.thebostonchannel.com/kelleys-story.

Elisha was diagnosed with breast cancer on the eve of her fortieth birthday in 2006, after finding a lump under her right arm. As she was not yet forty and had no history of cancer in her family, she, too, had never had a mammogram. After twenty-three mammogram images, doctors still could not see the lump that was clearly felt by touch. Elisha has small breasts, and the lump was far back under her arm. An ultrasound-guided biopsy confirmed that it was breast cancer. Further testing showed there was also lymph node involvement. After all her treatment options were presented to her, she and her doctor decided on a mastectomy, chemotherapy, hormone therapy, and radiation followed by reconstruction. Elisha is the fashion director for a Boston-based clothing designer and returned to work days after her mastectomy. She continued a busy schedule, including travel, throughout her treatment.

We were acquaintances before we were diagnosed who became close friends as we supported each other through treatment and beyond. We also shared a doctor at the Dana-Farber Cancer Institute in Boston. Dr. Ann Partridge is a wonderful oncologist who specializes in breast cancer in young women. We feel blessed to have such an amazing doctor and honored she agreed to serve as the medical editor for this book.

That said, this book is not intended to be a medical tome or replace your doctor's advice. We are here to share with you what helped us through treatment and perhaps provide some information that may spark good discussions with your medical providers. People will give you all sorts of advice on this journey, but every woman's experience is unique. You may find your road is a lot different, easier, or harder than ours. But we hope by reading this book you will remember you are not alone.

We agree that in many ways our lives are better than they were before cancer. We have friends whom we never would have met if we hadn't gotten sick. We have an inner strength that comes from facing an enormous challenge and overcoming it. We know the humbling, overwhelming, wonderful feeling of true compassion and kindness that our families and friends showed us during our darkest days.

So we beg you to begin this journey believing you will be among the vast majority of women who get this disease and beat it. We are here to help with the knowledge we have acquired in our own battles against this dreaded disease.

Shock and Awe

earing a doctor say you have cancer is a terrifying experience. Even when cancer runs in the family, this news usually comes as a shock. It's perfectly okay to spend some time feeling sorry for yourself. This is horribly upsetting news, and there's no reason why it should have happened to you. But it did.

It's important to realize that you are not responsible for this diagnosis. It's not your fault. It's not what you ate or didn't eat. Or the deodorant you use. Or the exercise equipment you never used. Scientists are still trying to figure out why some of us get this disease despite our best efforts to care for our bodies. It truly is a waste of time and energy to fret over "Why me?"

You may experience sleepless nights struggling with a mind that wants to go to those dark places, those worst-case scenarios. But you must keep telling yourself that you can do this. You can beat this disease. Try not to worry about death; focus on what you have to do to get well.

A diagnosis like this is sure to bring up thoughts of death, perhaps for the first time in your life. The hard truth is that we are all going to die, and most of us will not know the time or the cause. You have a challenge ahead of you that requires you to focus on treating and beating the disease, and focusing on death is contrary to your mission of getting well. Seek out examples all around you of people who faced enormous odds and beat them. Lance Armstrong comes to mind as a source of inspiration. Anything is possible.

After your diagnosis, you may be sent for further tests. You may need to have a biopsy. That may be followed by scans of your bones and organs to see if your cancer has spread beyond the breast. This is an unbelievably stressful time. You will literally have to stop your regularly scheduled life and devote yourself to doctors' appointments. It is very unsettling, and you may feel you have no control over your life anymore.

ELISHA: Those first days after your diagnosis are filled with sheer terror. The fear of the unknown is worse than facing any difficult reality. All the dreadful scenarios you imagine are enough to give you a huge mind cramp. Believe me—I know I dreamed up all sorts of horrible outcomes. The hardest thing for me to wrap my head around was the fact that this could happen to me. I liked to think that up to that moment, I had lived a very charmed life. I had been blessed with wonderful health, never spent a day in the hospital, never broken a bone, hardly ever had a head cold. All of a sudden, out of nowhere, I was just another statistic. Instead of fighting to get on the list for the latest Chanel bag, I was gearing up for the fight of my life.

I have spent most of my life in the fashion business in one capacity or another. For the past nine years, I have been the fashion director for a women's clothing designer in Boston. My job, along with my husband, family, and friends, has always consumed my life. The day I received my breast cancer diagnosis, the very first thing I thought about was the fact that I did not have time for this disruption in my life. My career requires me to travel extensively, and I was just about to get on a plane for Dallas and Atlanta. Instead, I was sent out on the battery of tests and doctors' appointments that follow your diagnosis.

LEARNING TO COPE

It's important to develop some coping strategies as soon as possible. While she was in those scan machines, Kelley used to sing Helen Reddy's "I Am Woman" to herself. By singing an empowering song, she could keep her mind focused on something other than the anxiety of the scan. She also brought headphones into her biopsy and listened to Aretha Franklin as the radiologist and her team worked. Kelley just needed a way to block out everything that was going on around her with a relaxing distraction.

No matter how much support you have in your life, there are places, such as scan machines, that you must go into alone. This is a time to develop your inner strength. Prayer carries many women through these dark hours. Other women may practice or learn meditation. Quite simply, you need to find a way to replace those dark thoughts with something positive and life affirming. Try repeating to yourself "I know I can do this" or "Anything is possible" or "I will get better!"

GOOD COMPANY

You will also learn quickly who makes you feel calm and safe and who makes you feel scared and sad. Be selfish and stick with friends and family who are best suited to helping you get through these difficult days. You cannot worry about hurting anyone's feelings; you have to take care of yourself. If you have an iPod, keep it handy. Music is a great distraction from the loneliness of hospital waiting rooms. If you have time, sneak out to see a funny movie. Your brain needs a distraction from thinking about cancer 24/7. Have a plan for what you will do at 2 a.m. if you cannot sleep. Keep a light fiction book or a funny DVD handy.

It's important to talk to your doctor if your anxiety feels overwhelming or is seriously affecting your ability to sleep or function. Kelley asked for sleeping pills during those first horrible days when every thought centered on the possibility of death and every night was sleepless. It's difficult to make good decisions about care when you are sleep deprived. You need rest to be able to cope with all that you have to do early in diagnosis. Don't be shy about talking to a doctor if you are struggling.

You can also ask your doctor to give you a referral to a social worker who has experience helping cancer patients and their families. He or she can help you cope with all the challenges you are facing now. You may also want to consider joining a support group so you can connect with other women. Your cancer center or the local American Cancer Society office can help you find one.

Spreading the News

You need to think about how and when you are going to let those around you know about this diagnosis. Decide how much you want people to know. We know of one woman who did not want her colleagues to know about her diagnosis. She continued to work through treatment and shared her experience only after it was all over. We all have to choose what's best for ourselves. We all have to find our own ways to cope.

Telling loved ones and coworkers can be an emotionally draining process. In some cases you may find it easier to ask a trusted friend or family member to communicate the news to people. Hearing their upset reactions simply may be too much to take.

Prepare yourself for the crazy things nervous people say. Cancer often makes people feel uncomfortable, and they will say anything that comes to mind. They may suggest a treatment that they know about, and you could stress out because your doctor never mentioned it. (Maybe that's because it's not appropriate for you!) Or they may recount a story about someone else's cancer saga even if it resulted in death. That's definitely not the most comforting thing to say to a newly diagnosed patient. People are trying to connect and empathize, but often it doesn't go so well.

So what are you going to do when someone starts in on a horrific story? Feel free to say, "How does this story end?" Tell the person you're not sure you can handle a sad story right now. If it's good news, let them go ahead. A little inspiration never hurt anyone. You can always come up with some sort of waving-off gesture to discourage long cancer stories. Pretend you're feeling nausea even if you haven't started chemo yet! They don't know. You have cancer—you can get away with being slightly rude to protect your emotional well-being.

ELISHA: Once my husband, Doug, and I absorbed the reality of my situation, we had to face the task of telling our family and friends. Telling my parents about my diagnosis was one of the hardest things I've ever done. It was so important for me to protect and comfort them, but I had to be honest and realistic.

I have no children, but I was very much married to my job. One of the first people I told about my diagnosis was my boss. I knew I was going to need her support and understanding to get through this with the least amount of disruption. I was fortunate that she embraced my situation, although I know she thought it would affect my responsibilities.

Doctor shopping, research, and appointments are very time consuming. You will wish you could be with your family and friends, or at work. I think it is important to keep your mind occupied with your normal routine whenever possible. I was at my best when I was at work during the day. Nights were always the hardest, because my mind would wander and I would beat myself up about how this happened to me. It took me a long time to get past the "Why me?" syndrome. I finally learned that I would never really know the answer to that question, and I was wasting precious time dwelling on it. I quickly decided in my heart and mind that this diagnosis would never define me. I was never going to be a cancer victim. I was Elisha Daniels, and I had many things to accomplish.

Now I had to convince my friends! I learned the hard way that telling friends about the diagnosis and accepting their sympathy can be overwhelming. I found myself telling the same frightening saga over and over again. I don't know

> how my coworkers put up with listening to me on the phone with well wishers every day. I began to feel like a broken record and quickly got sick of listening to my own story. For me, work was a place where I could concentrate on designing and merchandising our clothing line and not being a cancer patient. I tried very hard to keep my two worlds separate.

So what's the lesson here? We all need support and want others to feel compassion for us. As you get stronger, you may be better able to protect yourself emotionally. Elisha probably should have asked Doug to tell the story to some friends. Kelley probably should have told someone at work to spread the word that she was feeling positive and optimistic. Anyone who wanted to stop by and visit with her was welcome, but no "sad Sallys" allowed! You can order people to be positive or get lost. Really, you can. This is a fragile time emotionally, and you have to think of yourself first. You just do.

TALKING TO KIDS

Except, of course, if you have children at home. Then you have to think of them first. Dealing with children and their needs and fears is one of the most difficult parts of the cancer experience. For moms of children living at home, you immediately fear what would happen to them if you don't make it. You worry about their emotional well-being and day-to-day care. But, keep in mind, those should be adult worries for you and your partner. Have discussions privately away from little ears when you are sharing your concerns. Then agree on how you want to approach the kids and have a family talk. Try to pull it together and let your children see your strength.

You know your kids best and will know what they can handle. It's important to be truthful and straightforward while realizing they are not adults and may need to be protected from some of the news, depending on their ages. The experts suggest you use the correct terms such as cancer, not "boo boo." If a child asks you if you are going to die, try something such as, "My doctors and I have a plan to get Mom better, and we have every reason to believe it will be successful."

Kids tend to be self-centered and want to know how all this will affect them. You must assure them that they will be cared for at all times. In many cases, less information may be better. The best advice is to follow your kids' lead. If they are asking questions, by all means try to answer them. If they seem ready to move on, it's not necessary to drag out the conversation.

Throughout the process, asking them questions about what they are thinking and feeling is usually the best way to gauge if they are doing okay. Your hospital social worker and the American Cancer Society have more age-specific information that may help you talk to your children. And we have provided a lot more information and expert advice in chapter 10 if you want to skip ahead.

At some point, you or your partner will need to let the children's school know what's going on. Those can be difficult conversations. Kelley remembers breaking down in tears when she tried to let a pediatrician's nurse know she would not make an appointment. It brought up all those fears that she would not be able to care for her own children. Every call reminds you of how much your life has changed.

Most people are more than accommodating and want to help you and your family. Kelley had to remind people that she was not necessarily out for the count. She can remember showing up at school activities during treatment and having people look surprised. It was as if they were wondering, "What are you doing out of bed?" When you share the news with people, remind them that many cancer patients lead active lives despite treatment and that you will attend kids' activities as your health allows. People still have a perception that cancer means death or that treatment means you will be bedridden all the time. We can tell you firsthand neither of those misconceptions are true.

Sanity Saver

When you are ready, consider connecting with another woman who had a similar cancer at your stage of life. The American Cancer Society Reach to Recovery program (http://www.cancer.org or 800-227-2345) matches newly diagnosed patients with survivors. You can also ask friends if they know anyone. It usually makes it less scary to talk to someone who lived to tell the story!

LEARNING A NEW LANGUAGE

Kelley's husband, Brendan, put it well: "Getting a cancer diagnosis is like getting dropped off in a foreign country where you don't speak the language." There's a lot to learn about this complicated disease. Only you can decide how much you want to know. The Internet can be a scary place, and statistics can lead to sleepless nights. Proceed with caution. If you do want to go there, we have listed some great Web sites at the end of this book that we found to be most helpful.

It's probably a good idea that you understand some basic characteristics about your breast cancer. First, what type do you have? Noninvasive (or in situ) cancers are confined to the ducts or lobules and have not spread to the surrounding breast tissues or other parts of the body. Invasive cancers have started to break through to surrounding areas.

You will want to learn a few others things about your cancer, but most won't be known until after surgery:

Tumor size

Tumor grade (a measure of tumor aggressiveness, rated from one to three, with three being the most aggressive)

Axillary lymph node status (Are nodes involved? If so, how many?)

Hormone receptor status (Is your cancer sensitive to estrogen and progesterone?)

HER2/neu status (Does your cancer overexpress this protein, which is a mark of tumor aggressiveness but can be targeted with special treatment, such as with Herceptin?)

These will all play a role in what you can expect in terms of treatment. Your education begins with Dr. Partridge's Breast Cancer 101:

Breast cancer can be a local (e.g., breast, chest wall, axilla/underarm area) and systemic disease (potential for cells spreading elsewhere in the body). From a local standpoint, the surgeon tries to cut it all out both in the breast and in the lymph nodes. Unfortunately, though, cells can escape from the area where the cancer mass is locally, and some women need radiation for additional local treatment. From a systemic standpoint, cells may also escape not only locally in the breast tissue, if any, chest, and underarm area, but elsewhere in the body. If these cells are able to grow back and form tumor masses, this is called recurrent, and often metastatic, breast cancer (meaning it has spread elsewhere beyond the chest and axilla, or underarm). Breast cancer that has spread is generally incurable and what all of the treatments that you will consider are trying to prevent.

It is your doctors' job to not only remove the cancer locally, but to also use the features of your cancer and your unique circumstances to estimate the chances that cells may have escaped either locally or systemically and to help you to determine which treatments are worth the risks they entail to reduce the chances that you will hear from your cancer again. At different points in your treatment you will learn about potential side effects you may encounter. These can be quite serious but are usually rare. Make sure you fully discuss the potential risks and benefits of each treatment including chemotherapy and/or hormonal therapy with your caregivers.

You may also hear or ask doctors about what stage they consider your cancer. That is a number from one to four, with four being the most advanced. A word about staging: It may be good to know where you fit on the spectrum, but don't become obsessed with this or any number. There are amazing treatments available today, and many women are living long lives after being diagnosed with cancers in all stages.

Here's some great advice from a doctor who knows the emotional roller coaster of cancer all too well: "Try not to get too excited about news you perceive to be good or too upset about news you perceive to be negative."

That proved to be helpful advice for Kelley, whose postsurgery pathology report showed four positive lymph nodes, advancing the diagnosis from stage two to stage three cancer. Six months later, when doctors reviewed the pathology in preparation for radiation treatment, they found one lymph node had been counted twice. It was stage two all along.

Try to keep your feelings about all these numbers and statistics in check. You are an individual, not a statistic.

Don't Lose Your Sanity!

- Believe you can beat this!
- Try exercise, yoga, or meditation to clear your mind.
- Distract yourself with books and movies.
- Surround yourself with people who make you feel better.
- Talk to your doctor if you find anxiety overwhelming or are having trouble sleeping. Medication may help.

Don't Lose Your Style!

- Send a message to the world that you are healing, not dying!
- Try to stick to your routine when possible. Go to work. Take the kids to school. You can still be you, not a patient all the time.
- Pamper yourself—get a massage, a facial, or a manicure.
- Keep wearing makeup—everyone will be looking for signs of your decline.
- Throw on your high heels—we all look better in heels!

Go Team!

*g*oing to a wedding? You probably would go to a few stores to find the perfect dress. Remodeling the bathroom? You wouldn't dream of not getting at least two estimates. Going to have major surgery? I'll just go with what he or she says. Are you sure?

Perhaps you are convinced you have the best doctor already, but there is nothing wrong with getting a second opinion after being diagnosed. In fact, we strongly encourage it. Different doctors and different institutions may have varying takes on the best course of treatment. We certainly know that doctors have different styles, and you may simply "click" better with one than another.

Did your mother ever tell you "You are only as good as the company you keep"? The team of doctors you assemble to guide you through this journey may be the most important decision you will ever make. We are fortunate to live in Boston, a city full of some of the best doctors and hospitals in the world, but we still had to do our homework.

Who's Who

You may need several different doctors over the course of your treatment. Most people will need a surgeon to either perform a lumpectomy or a mastectomy. Your medical oncologist will oversee the bulk of your treatment and care. Choose this doctor carefully, because you two will likely be seeing each other for several years! Most of us will undergo radiation treatment, so you will also need a radiation oncologist who will be responsible for seeing you through that part of the journey. You should also consider meeting with a plastic surgeon so you know all the options for reconstruction as early as possible. That meeting was key for Kelley, who learned that her reconstruction could take place at the same time as her mastectomy. You may also want to consider meeting with a physical therapist if your surgery may affect your range of motion.

Kelley found the process of "doctor shopping" extremely empowering at a time when she could barely function.

KELLEY: I met my surgeon through a referral from my ob-gyn. This amazing woman was there for me the day I was diagnosed and immediately made me feel comfortable and safe. I trusted her implicitly. I knew she had both the experience and the bedside manner to get me through my mastectomy, so I didn't want to get a second opinion. It made the whole thing feel too real, and I just wanted to get treatment over with! But my family and friends nearly forced me to go see other doctors. I had friends calling me to say they had already set up the appointment if I would just go. That was really helpful, because I was somewhat paralyzed at that point. I really did not have it together at all. I was terrified.

With each visit, I learned more about my disease and treatment options. It suddenly felt like I was getting my mojo back after being knocked to the ground by the diagnosis. Visiting doctors and taking charge of my own care was empowering. You also learn you are far from the only person stuck with this hideous disease. Friends and acquaintances recommended Dr. Partridge, an oncologist whose style and bedside manner made me feel instantly like I was with a trusted friend. As soon as I met her, I knew she was the one I wanted to guide me on this journey. I stuck with my original surgeon whom I instinctively trusted, but those second opinions confirmed my initial feelings.

My choices of doctors meant I would have my surgery at one hospital and treatment at another. That was my preference, and the institutions seemed more than willing to accommodate me. I was suddenly a woman with a plan, and I was starting to feel stronger and less afraid.

TAKE YOUR TIME

Dr. Partridge says, "Breast cancer is an emotional emergency, but usually not a medical emergency." What does that mean? It means you have time to research your options. You have time to find the right doctors for you. But she acknowledges that this is a very difficult time for a woman and her family. Dr. Partridge calls it the "limbo period," when a woman does not know what she has or what she needs to do about it. It's often the most difficult and anxiety-producing time. She reassures her patients that they will feel better once there's a plan and they are moving forward with it.

ELISHA: I felt so blessed that I fell into the amazing hands of my breast surgeon, who performed my mastectomy at Massachusetts General Hospital. He has a long list of amazing credentials, but just as important, he was kind and thoughtful. He seemed to understand all that I was going through both physically and mentally. That made a huge difference, because inside I was a nervous wreck and completely overwhelmed by the decisions I felt unqualified to make.

I'm a huge proponent of taking your medical care into your own hands. Do your own research and shop around for the best doctor who fits your needs. These people are going to be in your life for a long time, so you need to be crazy about them.

Trust Your Gut

When it was time for Elisha to pick a medical oncologist, she knew it was an important decision because this doctor would probably be the one she would consult for years to come. But when she met with the medical oncologist at the cancer center, she had a difficult time feeling comfortable. There was no bond. She tried to ignore her feelings and kept telling herself he had impressive credentials.

Still, that nagging feeling of uncertainty would not go away, so Elisha sought out other options. Two friends recommended she meet with Dr. Partridge. Like Kelley, Elisha found her to be a much better fit.

Doctor Shopping

So how do you find those other options? Start by asking any of your current trusted physicians for recommendations. They refer patients to oncologists all the time, and they know the good ones. Do you have other friends or acquaintances in the medical field? They may know someone to recommend. Contact or ask someone else to get in touch with everyone you know who has survived breast cancer. Ask them for referrals. This is a great job for someone who has offered to help you but doesn't know where to begin. They can check out doctors for you.

Sanity Saver

Get organized! You will have a lot of paperwork and a lot of information to process. Consider getting a three-ring binder. Punch holes in all those medical reports so you will know where to find them. Get a notebook for note taking at your various appointments. Keep your doctors' phone numbers on the inside page so you can find them easily.

BRING ALONG A SECOND SET OF EARS

When you go for your second opinion, try to take the same person who came with you to your first appointment. That way you will have another person with whom you can share notes and impressions. It is so difficult to process everything the doctors and nurses are saying to you. We can't stress enough how important it is to have a trusted person in the room to help you digest it all. We've even heard of people tape recording a session with their doctor so they can play it over again once they're home. Obviously, check with the doctor to see if he or she is comfortable with the idea, but it's one way to make sure you're getting all the key information. You will certainly have lots of questions, so consider carrying a little notebook with you at all times to write them down. You can also type them into your PDA. Then bring those questions with you to appointments so you won't forget to ask something important!

You will know you've found the right caregiver when you find a doctor you can trust and have confidence in his or her abilities. You should feel comfortable enough to express concerns, ask questions, and make sure you understand the answers. You may also find a good fit with someone who has a specialty in your particular cancer, such as triple negative, HER2/neu positive, or genetic cancers.

At some cancer centers you will meet all of these doctors on one day, either all together or one after another. It can definitely be an overwhelming experience. If your cancer center has a nurse coordinating the care or a cancer navigator, seek that person out. They are usually excellent guides through this challenging time.

KELLEY: I can still remember the day I had to go to the hospital for the meeting with all the doctors. I had it in my head we would all be sitting at a table and go over one plan. Instead they came in one after another until my head was spinning. One said we would do surgery first. The other said it might be chemo first. We still didn't have all the biopsy results in yet, so they really couldn't definitively give me a plan. It was so frustrating! It was my first taste of the wild ride that is the cancer experience. Every time you try to gain a little control, something happens to throw you off. There are many ups and downs. To me, the meet-the-doctors day was a real downer. I just couldn't believe everything they were saying. It seemed overwhelming how much treatment I would need. That was definitely a low point for me. I didn't feel stronger until I finally became motivated to get that second opinion.

WEIGHING YOUR OPTIONS

You may have few options for care in your area, or perhaps you're in an area of the country with a variety of options. A lot of people wonder whether it's better to get care at a big-city hospital or a community hospital closer to home. That's a difficult question to answer. The case for the big-city teaching hospitals may be obvious. You will have access to excellent care at institutions where ongoing research may be beneficial to your treatment. These big cancer centers often have excellent support programs and extras, such as yoga and acupuncture, on-site. But these can be busy, bustling places that are not easy to get to, particularly if you require frequent visits.

A comprehensive cancer center can actually design a treatment plan that can be administered at a hospital more conveniently located.

We asked Dr. Tim Moynihan, a medical oncologist at the prestigious Mayo Clinic, to answer some common questions about planning your cancer care.

Q: What's the best way for patients to find excellent surgeons and oncologists?

A: There are many well-trained and excellent surgeons, medical oncologists, and radiation oncologists throughout the country. I think the first place to start is with your primary physician. Whom do they recommend? Whom would they go to? How long have they been working with these physicians/facilities? Are the facilities up to date? Do they participate in clinical trials research? (This is often a sign that the group is at the leading edge of treatments. They can take place in small hospitals and communities; clinical trials are not confined to big cities or academic centers.) For the surgeons specifically: How often do they do the specific operation? How many patients with similar conditions do they care for? You do not want to have a very difficult or technical operation done by someone who does only one every few years. If your local surgeon is skilled and well trained but doesn't do many of your specific procedures, you will want to go to a referral center. On the other hand, if you have a common condition, the local surgeon may do many such operations and would be well qualified. For medical oncology and radiation: Participation in clinical trials is a good sign. For radiation, the facilities are important: Do they have up-to-date equipment? Ask your friends, relatives, and neighbors whom they have seen. Were the physicians receptive? Did they answer their questions, or were they hurried and never had time for the patient?

Q: **What should a patient consider when deciding whether to seek care in a suburban facility close to home or go to a big-city hospital?**

A: For most common presentations of common cancers, the local facility will be fine. The question is how do you know what you have is common—both the type of cancer as well as the specifics of your case? I would say, ask your primary doctor as well as the surgeons, medical oncologists, and radiation oncologists. Each patient is always unique, but is special expertise required in your circumstances? Is there something truly different or challenging about your specific case? If the answer is yes (for example, you have a rare tumor or a common cancer with unusual or challenging circumstances), then referral to a specialty center is reasonable. For all cancers, a one-time second opinion is always reasonable. If the experts say that the treatment at home would be just as good as here, then for the sake of convenience you might as well be treated at home.

Q: **Under which circumstances would you recommend a patient seek care at a nationally known facility such as the Mayo Clinic?**

A: For patients with unique or challenging circumstances in which highly specialized care is required, being seen at a nationally recognized center is appropriate. Perhaps special surgical therapy is required, or you may benefit from experimental, or "cutting-edge," treatments or technology. Again, a second opinion at a leading center is always reasonable. Most primary surgeons, medical oncologists, and radiation oncologists welcome the advice and opinions of the leading centers.

SEEK OUT OTHER RESOURCES

You may want to think about contacting the hospital's social worker at some point. This is someone who knows the drill and has guided other women through treatment. He or she can help you cope with the difficult emotional challenges you face, which at times can be worse than the physical challenges. Often you can schedule a meeting with a social worker while you are at the cancer center for another appointment. They can certainly help with family issues and empower you with the tools you need to get through this. They can also point you in the right direction for support groups or more intensive counseling if you need it.

CONTACT YOUR INSURER

You must get on the phone with your insurance company as soon as possible. Many companies have major illness case managers who will help you get through treatment with the maximum benefits possible. Pay close attention to finding in-network caregivers or getting necessary referrals. Treatment is going to be expensive enough without incurring unexpected medical costs. And definitely make sure you get your surgery and hospital stay preapproved—most plans require it.

Once you settle on a team, ask your doctors for the best way to contact them. Can you have their pager or cell phone numbers? Are they reachable by e-mail? Make sure you know their nurses' names and numbers, because they are often your best resources. Get to know the office schedules so you can plan appointments accordingly.

Once your team is in place, you will find yourself breathing a little easier. You still have a long road ahead of you, but at least now you know with whom you are dealing. You have doctors and nurses to answer your questions and help you guide you down the road to recovery.

Don't Lose Your Sanity

- Take a breath. You probably have time to find the right docs for you.
- Bring a trusted loved one to appointments to help you sort through the information and discuss the doctor's bedside manner.
- Get organized. Keep reports in one place, along with notes and important phone numbers.
- Consider meeting with a hospital social worker to sort through challenges and feelings.
- Don't worry if the rest of your life is falling apart. Once you pick a team and start treatment, you should be able to pull it together!

Don't Lose Your Style

- Go out to lunch or dinner with an old, trusted friend who will entertain you with topics other than cancer chat.
- Head out to a funny, feel-good movie.
- Retail therapy really does work. Buy a pair of shoes or a fabulous new lipstick color. Either one will give you a much-needed lift.
- Don't sweat the small stuff. Your life has suddenly become much too complicated to worry about small problems.
- Make time to meet with a plastic surgeon early on if you might be heading toward a mastectomy so you will know all your options. Surviving is the priority, but you want to know your options for putting yourself back together again.

THREE

Surgery

Surgery usually makes most people anxious. Cancer surgery makes people very anxious. You are not alone if it feels terrifying to put your life in a medical team's hands. It is scary. In fact, Kelley wrote a letter to her family the night before surgery just in case she didn't make it. Of course, there was no rational reason to believe she wouldn't come through it just fine. Which she did. Elisha remembers preparing for her mastectomy as the most frightening time in her life. The thought of going into surgery and not knowing what she would look like afterward was horrifying. She knew she would wake up disfigured, and that was simply overwhelming.

So how do you work through those feelings? Try to keep in mind that this is your opportunity to get the cancer out of your body. Repeat that over and over to yourself until you really believe it. Surgery is often your first step toward healing. Try to see it as something positive in your battle instead of a negative.

EXPECT THE UNEXPECTED

The most important thing to remember about surgery is that there may be some surprises when you wake up or later in your recovery. You have to be emotionally prepared for that possibility. For many women, the surgery will include a sentinel node biopsy to see if the cancer has spread to the lymph nodes. If it has spread, you may have to have lymph nodes removed. You may ultimately need chemotherapy, hormone therapy, and/or radiation therapy. If you weren't expecting this, the news can be devastating.

Go into surgery recognizing that something the surgeon finds may change your treatment plan. That's simply a frustrating part of this process. Breast cancer is not one disease, and it does not come with just one treatment plan. You may be about to learn that the hard way. After surgery you will likely get an even better sense of exactly what you are facing.

If you decide to undergo a lumpectomy, that can turn from one surgery into several. You will hear an expression called "clear margins," which refers to whether or not the entire tumor mass has been removed. If a surgeon does not get clear margins on the first surgery, he or she may have to go back in to remove more tissue. It can be very frustrating to hear you may need multiple surgeries, but, sadly, this is not uncommon. In some cases, lumpectomies can turn into mastectomies if the surgeon finds the disease is more widespread than anticipated.

A friend of ours recently went in for a lumpectomy and assumed it would be followed by radiation and hormone therapy. Unfortunately, during surgery the doctors found that the cancer had spread to the lymph nodes and she woke up to hear some disturbing news. She will now need chemotherapy. It is a tough way to recover but a very real possibility for many women. It's better to recognize the potential for changes in your treatment ahead of time so you won't be thrown off too much by unexpected news.

WHICH SURGERY IS RIGHT FOR YOU?

What type of local therapy to receive depends on both the extent of disease in the breast and your preferences and values regarding the pros and cons, if there are choices. Some women will have disease that encompasses much of the breast so that anything less than a mastectomy will not be a reasonable option. Many women will be offered the choice of a lumpectomy or a mastectomy. A lumpectomy is usually paired with radiation; this has been shown to be as good as a mastectomy in the long run, assuming both surgeries have removed the obvious disease in the breast. Every patient's situation is different, so deciding which surgery is best will require serious conversations with your doctors as well as thoughts about your preferences and values. Some women prefer to keep their natural breast if possible, while others will opt for a mastectomy. Some women choose to have reconstruction while others do not. You can ask both your surgeon and your medical oncologist to advise you. If you are undecided, or do not like the treatments offered to you, this is an excellent example of why a second opinion can be so vital. These experts can help guide you in your decision-making process.

For many women, choosing the type of surgery will be a wrenching decision. Take your time to make the right choices. This is essential for other decisions such as chemo or no chemo, radiation or no radiation. Talk to as many medical professionals as you can, talk to survivors, speak with a social worker, do your own research. Then talk with your loved ones and other trusted advisers and make the best decision you can.

KELLEY: I knew at diagnosis that at least one lymph node was involved. Later I found out there was disease in different parts of the breast, including one rather large tumor. Grim news indeed. It was clear to all the doctors who reviewed my case that I would require a mastectomy. I honestly did not focus too much on the loss of my breast. I knew I had a serious case, and I did not want to die. My husband told me he felt the exact same way. He would still love and be attracted to a woman who was surgically altered. We agreed the most important thing was survival. I came to peace with the mastectomy part of all this surprisingly fast. It was the cancer and the potential for death that had me really freaked out.

PROPHYLACTIC MASTECTOMIES

You often hear about women prophylactically removing the breast with no disease. How do you decide if that's the right option for you? Here's what Dr. Partridge tells her patients:

For most women, removal of the unaffected breast does not make sense, as it is not likely to help a woman improve her survival in the long run. Unless a woman has a high risk of a new primary breast cancer occurring in that breast over the next several years (for example, she is a BRCA1 or BRCA2 mutation carrier, or has received radiation to her chest for lymphoma as a young person), removal of the other breast is generally not indicated. We have to be careful to counsel women not to remove body parts unnecessarily to treat anxiety. There are other, better treatments for anxiety.

GENETIC TESTING

That, of course, brings up the question of whether you should be tested for the BRCA gene. Five to ten percent of breast cancer patients will have a hereditary form of the disease. Two genes have been discovered, which, when altered, increase a woman's susceptibility for developing breast and ovarian cancer. These genes are called BRCA1 and BRCA2, and they are located on chromosome 17 and 13, respectively. Human cells contain two sets of chromosomes (organized structures of DNA and protein). One set is inherited from the mother and one is inherited from the father, and each set contains twenty-three single chromosomes. A genetic mutation, or change in the DNA segment, on the BRCA1 or BRCA2 gene is associated with a 50 to 85 percent chance of developing breast cancer over the course of a woman's lifetime.

You should ask your doctor about testing if:

- You have a family history of multiple cases of breast cancer or cases of both breast and ovarian cancer, particularly if diagnosed at young ages.
- One or more of your family members had two primary cancers.
- You are of Ashkenazi (eastern European) Jewish background.
- You are under age 40 when diagnosed with breast cancer.

This is a test you must discuss with your doctor and your insurance company. It's a pricey blood test done at only one lab in the country. You will want to make sure your insurance covers it before you get stuck with a several-thousand-dollar bill. You will also want to meet with a genetic counselor at your hospital so you can be prepared for the results. A positive test result may change the treatment plan, as these patients have a greater risk of both breast and ovarian cancer.

Preparing for Surgery

Before you go into the hospital, come up with a plan for how work and home will run without you. Talk to your employer about what you expect in terms of recovery, but be honest and tell your supervisor that the plan may change. Make arrangements for your children and reassure them that their routine will continue as always. Don't forget pets! Ask a trusted family member or friend to help coordinate household activities while you are hospitalized.

KELLEY: Believe it or not, I had a massage the night before my mastectomy. My sister was sweet enough to whisk me away to a spa that Sunday afternoon, and then we joined the family at my house for dinner that night. It wasn't the best massage I've ever had because I could not really relax. But it certainly didn't hurt! I was just sick of the build-up and eager to get the surgery over with. My mother was crying as I left for the hospital that morning and said she would do anything to trade places with me. I knew she meant it, and I was deeply touched. But I also told her to pull it together because I needed her to be strong for me. I had it in my head I could do this and that I would be tumor free on the other side. I was determined to get cancer behind me, and surgery was my first step.

Kelley went to the hospital with her husband, Brendan, and her father. Kelley's mom watched the kids and kept the routine as normal as possible. Elisha would only allow her husband, Doug, to come to the hospital. She simply could not take responsibility for comforting anyone else in her devastated family.

We have both learned you have to do what works best for you. You can't worry about what anyone else is feeling right now. Just focus on what makes you feel better. It truly is the one time in your life where being self-ish is okay. The only exception, of course, is if you have children at home. Then you will want to take care in how you handle your hospitalization and visits.

Kelley did like having friends and family around to keep the mood light, and she did have her then nearly three-year-old come in for one visit. They brought in a DVD player so Kelley and Maddie could cuddle in the hospital bed and watch a movie. That allowed them to be physically close in a way that didn't exhaust or hurt Kelley's sore body. The baby did not come to the hospital for several reasons, and Kelley is still okay with that decision. You know your kids and what they can handle. This is a decision you can make after you see how you feel postsurgery. Just be honest and straightforward with the kids and tell them you will talk to them after surgery and come up with a plan for how and when they will see you.

ELISHA: Despite my trauma over going in for surgery, in the back of my mind, I was also worried about how I was going to look when I came out. The Saturday before surgery, I had a manicure and pedicure. I had my manicurist cut my fingernails off so the medical staff could easily put on the pulse monitor. That's a small machine that clips onto your finger to keep track of your pulse. Nurses usually tell you not to wear nail polish to surgery so it won't interfere with the monitor. But I had my toenails painted bright red. There was no way I was going to lie on an operating table or wake up in a cold hospital bed without pretty toes. That's just me! But, most important, it made me feel like I still had some control over how I looked, and that made me feel better.

When you arrive at the hospital you will have to answer a lot of questions over and over again. Get used to it! The key is to make sure they know why you are there and that they do not remove the wrong breast! You'll find they check which side a lot.

The Surgery

Both of us remember being fairly out of it as we were being wheeled down those long hospital corridors. Elisha remembers thinking how cold and sterile it was in the operating room. A friend had prepared Kelley for the crosslike shape of the table and how, as a Catholic, she found that somewhat disturbing. Fortunately, you will quickly fall asleep and let the capable medical caregivers do what they need to do to make you well.

ELISHA: In the end, surgery is the easiest part of the whole process. They put you to sleep, you take a nap, and you come out clean and new. It is ultimately so wonderfully liberating to know the nasty cancer tumor has been taken out of you. I knew having my breast removed was the first step to moving on with the rest of my life.

When I woke up in the recovery room, the first thing I asked for was my lipstick. I know that might sound crazy to you, but I wanted to look my best when my husband came in to see me. I fluffed my hair, put on my lipstick, put a smile on my face, and greeted him like I was meeting him for the first time. I was so happy and so grateful. I felt this huge sense of accomplishment that I had survived this round. Remember, girls, that which you survive will make you stronger.

One word—preapproval! Take the time to get as much of your care preapproved as possible. Check out the doctors, even anesthesiologists, to see if they are covered by your insurance plan. If any proposed treatment seems experimental or different from widely accepted protocol, talk to your insurance plan first. We have heard horror stories of women being stuck with huge bills for even such things as radiation because the insurance company deemed the type they received experimental. These cases are rare but are something to consider.

SURVEYING THE DAMAGE

At some point you will have to open the surgical dressings and take a look at the damage. It's okay to mourn what you have lost, because it's not easy to have your body changed so drastically. But, remember, this is just the beginning and there are ways to get you looking more like yourself again. For many of us the goal is simply to look good and natural in our clothes. For others the thought of a partner seeing us naked again is terrifying. We urge you to take this one step at a time. Right now the most important thing is to recover physically from this surgery.

If you have had a mastectomy or lymph nodes removed, you will notice your breast, underarm, and shoulder area feel different. A mastectomy incision, reconstruction, and underarm area can all lose sensation. You may have a breast through reconstruction, but, unfortunately, it will not be sensitive to touch any longer. And you need to be careful when shaving under your arm, because you will likely not feel the razor. You may never need to shave under that arm again. The hair might just not grow back.

Postsurgery

So what do you need postsurgery? You may want to have some button, snap, or tie-on tops that are easy to get on and off, because you might have difficulty putting your arms over your head. There are some products available with a handy pocket for the drain or drains you will need to wear for the next few days. A company called Healing Threads makes a stylish line of postsurgery clothes with easy access and drain pockets. You can also use safety pins to attach drains to the inside of your current clothes.

There's no rule that says you have to wear those horrible hospital johnnies during your recovery. You can usually wear what you want as long as the doctors and nurses have easy access to your incisions and drains.

Down the Drain

Many of us get a little squeamish about the drains. They are usually coming out of your underarms so fluid does not build up, and they are a little gross. Fortunately, you won't have to wear them too long, and they are relatively easy to maintain. You may want to consider having a visiting nurse stop by when you are at home just to check the drains and make sure you are healing right. Check to see if your insurance plan will cover this type of visit.

Restoring Range of Motion

Postsurgery, consider going to physical therapy to help restore the full range of motion in your arm or arms if it's an issue. In fact, some physical therapists believe you should visit them before the surgery so they can examine you and get a better sense of how the surgery has affected you. The hospital, your surgeon, or your physical therapist can give you a list of exercises to do postsurgery. You may feel a strange "cording," or axillary web syndrome, under your arm(s). This is like a web of tightness that emanates from the scar tissue or radiated areas and feels like cords. Some PTs can do manual therapy or suggest exercises to ease or eliminate cording.

We can remember getting out of the hospital and attempting to do our "snow angel" exercises and not being able to move our arms past our shoulders. It's very frustrating and scary. But the only way you will get your range of motion back is to do your exercises.

You do not have to accept limitations from your cancer treatment. Physical therapy may help you get back to enjoying activities you liked before treatment. It was also supportive to have a trained professional guide us through the recovery and help measure our progress. This is one part of the cancer journey where you don't passively sit back and receive treatment.

The doctors and nurses are here to help save your life, but a physical therapist may help restore the quality of your life. To find someone in your area who has experience dealing with breast cancer patients go to the American Physical Therapy Association's Web site at http://www.apta.org. There you can search for a PT with experience in oncology.

LYMPHEDEMA

You will also want to be aware of and take precautions against lymphedema, a chronic swelling condition that women can be at risk for if they have had lymph nodes removed. There's no exact formula for why certain people will have a problem, and you may get a lot of confusing information about this condition. Risk factors include greater extent of axillary surgery, being overweight, and having radiation.

Nancy Roberge is a physical therapist who specializes in breast cancer survivors. Because there is so little medical data available, she has developed some unofficial guidelines for her patients to assess risk that you may find helpful. She cautions that this is based on anecdotal information rather than scientific evidence.

Low risk: Three to four lymph nodes or fewer removed and no radiation

Medium risk: Multiple lymph nodes removed and no radiation

High risk: Multiple positive lymph nodes with radiation

Roberge points out that you can be at risk for lymphedema for the rest of your life. Many of her patients experience swelling years after breast cancer treatment.

Studies have not proven what exactly causes lymphedema or how to avoid it. However, Roberge does suggest the following steps you can take to reduce the chances of getting lymphedema, based on her years of experience with women:

- Avoid heavy lifting.
- Avoid needle pricks and blood pressure cuffs on your affected side.
- Try not to carry heavy bags on your affected side.
- Try to avoid burns or cuts on your affected side. If you do get them, treat them quickly with antibiotics. Use sunscreen.
- Don't allow a manicurist to cut the cuticles on your affected arm to avoid infections.
- Some experts believe spending time in a Jacuzzi or sauna may cause or exacerbate swelling.

Roberge does have some dos as well:

- Wear a compression sleeve when flying and doing repetitive, strenuous activity. Your surgeon should be able to refer you to where you can get a sleeve and write you a prescription so insurance will pay for it. We bought ours at the hospital oncology shop. There's also a Web site called LympheDivas (http://lymphedivas.com) that sells much more stylish versions!
- Swimming is useful in decreasing lymphedema.

- Deep breathing encourages lymph flow and helps you relax.
- Drinking six to eight glasses of water a day can help with lymph drainage and lessen fluid retention.

If you start to notice swelling on your affected arm or if it starts to feel unusually heavy, get in touch with your surgeon or physical therapist. There are steps they can take to minimize the swelling. If your arm becomes red, painful, warm, and/or swollen, this may be a sign of an infection that may require immediate medical care.

ELISHA: My radiation oncologist put a lot of emphasis on lymphedema and rightfully so; many women suffer from this challenging side effect. I was very disturbed by this condition and did everything I could to prevent it. One of the first things I did was work with a professional physical therapist, who helped me regain my full range of motion in my arm and shoulder after my mastectomy. I also followed my doctor's orders and wore a sleeve every time I got on a plane. Okay—let's chat about this a minute. I'm a total fashionista and this sleeve is definitely not the hottest look off the Paris runway. The best way I can describe it to you is that it's like a tight girdle for your arm. However, I am on a plane going somewhere almost once a week, and I wear my sleeve regularly and have never had any problems. I also avoid carrying heavy bags on my affected side. I promise you, you will feel the consequences. I remember being in Atlanta at a fashion show a few weeks after my mastectomy, and just picking clothes up and down off a rolling rack made my affected side completely swell up. Lesson learned! Listen to your body.

Bouncing Back

It's never easy to go from a robust life to being bedridden or at least housebound. It's hard to give up so much control over your body and your life. The doctors, nurses, and others who work in oncology tend to be the most amazing caregivers. We wouldn't be alive if it weren't for their skill, compassion, and support. But being in the hospital is not easy. People tend to come into your room at all hours, and it's unnerving. Getting sleep seems impossible even though that's what you really need. In the hospital you'll want to stay on top of matters related to your care or ask someone you love to do it. There's been a lot of talk about how long women can stay in the hospital following a mastectomy. Kelley put her foot down when she felt she was being rushed out the door.

KELLEY: I mostly had an excellent experience at the hospital, but it wasn't perfect. You will have some nurses who are amazing and make you feel so secure. But I did have a few who did not seem to understand the procedure I just had. I woke up to a nurse putting a cuff on my right mastectomy arm, and I freaked out. After that I asked for a sign above my bed and a ribbon on my arm saying no blood pressure on that side. After two nights of hospitalization they wanted to send me home. My surgery included major reconstruction in addition to a mastectomy. I still had a pain pump in me and was going home to a two-year-old and baby. I put my foot down. I know they like to get you out of the hospital because the risk for infection is greater there, but I decided to take my chances. It was too hard for me to go home before I was ready.

When you are ready, home is a nicer place to recover. You should just plan to take it easy, recognizing that you've been through a lot. If people offer to help, accept it! You need to focus on getting well.

For Elisha that meant getting back to work as quickly as possible.

ELISHA: I had my mastectomy on a Wednesday morning, went home on Friday afternoon, and I went back to work the next Monday. I had no interest in staying in the hospital one minute more than necessary. My doctor made sure I was well wrapped and bandaged, and I decided I would be better off recovering at home with the assistance of a visiting nurse. I had two drains under my right arm, which definitely took time to get used to. I had to learn to empty and strip them a few times a day. They were cumbersome and bulky under my fabulous outfits, but mostly they completely grossed me out. I remember going out to dinner with Doug that Friday night to our favorite little pizza place around the corner from our home, and I was afraid to have a glass of wine because I thought it might come out through my drains. Is this the craziest thought you've ever heard? Well, believe me; you will have some crazy thoughts, too. And that's okay. Like any new experience, you learn as you go along.

The day my bandages were scheduled to come off was another scary day for me. My nurse came to my house, and we did it together. I stood in front of a long mirror in my bedroom and prepared myself for what I thought would be a gruesome sight. What I saw was certainly unbalanced, let's say, but definitely not gruesome. I knew once all my treatment was over, I would have reconstruction and end up with the boobs I had always wanted. The thought of reconstruction ended up being my carrot, or shall we say my Jimmy Choos, at the end of a long, difficult road.

So try to face this first step of cancer treatment with courage and confidence. You have to believe you are on your way to getting better.

Don't Lose Your Sanity!

- Pick a great surgeon and trust him or her!
- Convince yourself that surgery is an opportunity to get well, not something to fear.
- Resume a normal life as soon as you are able. Go out to dinner or a movie, and go back to work. Do what you feel capable of doing. It will make you feel like yourself again.
- Seek physical therapy to regain full range of motion.
- Accept help after surgery so you can focus on healing.

Don't Lose Your Style!

- Pick out a beautiful nightgown or top to wear in the hospital or at home postsurgery.
- Get out your oversized sweaters and jackets to cover up your drains.
- Wear lipstick and toenail polish to your mastectomy!
- Talk to your hair stylist about getting a new, fresh short haircut before chemotherapy begins.
- Attitude is everything, and you can still be fabulous with two, one, or no boobs!

Reconstruction and Prosthetics

reconstruction is something you may want to consider if a mastectomy is part of your treatment plan. But it is certainly not a medical or emotional necessity. This is a personal decision you can absolutely make on your own once you've considered all options. Dr. Partridge says reconstruction is not believed to affect the risk of recurrence or the ability to detect a recurrence or a new primary breast cancer.

Most women who have a lumpectomy do not have plastic surgery even though the cosmetic results may not be ideal. But Dr. Stephanie Caterson, a plastic surgeon at Brigham and Women's Hospital in Boston, says there are some options for patients who have undergone lumpectomy and radiation, so consider getting a consultation if you are unhappy with your posttreatment appearance.

You can also look into enhancers, which are partial breast forms you place in your bra to match your other breast. They are available in oncology or specialty shops.

Talk to a Plastic Surgeon ASAP

It's best to think about reconstruction options as early as possible. Only a plastic surgeon can tell you for sure what's possible. But then you need to run any plans by your oncologist to make sure the reconstruction won't interfere with the treatment. In some cases, radiation can limit your options and/or your timing. You may need to discuss your unique situation with a plastic surgeon and your radiation oncologist.

Like many decisions along the breast cancer road, you will need to weigh the pros and cons of having reconstruction, as well as the type and timing of plastic surgery. And, as we've mentioned, you don't need to do it. In some cases you may not be a good candidate for reconstruction for medical reasons. It really depends on your preferences and values.

You certainly don't need to do reconstruction right away, although your options may be more limited by waiting. Dr. Caterson says delaying your reconstruction can also change the scar pattern on your chest, as the plastic surgeon will have less skin to work with if you've already had your mastectomy. You can choose to wait until you feel more prepared to handle another surgery, or you may have to wait until you finish treatment because of safety concerns. Getting the picture here? Reconstruction is like the rest of this crazy journey. Lots of different possibilities, but each person may ultimately have few or many options! Having fun yet?

Consider Your Options

We suggest you consider all your options early and then make the best decision you can, given all that's going on in your life right now. Dr.

Caterson provided us with a look at what's available right now in terms of reconstruction. She was Elisha's surgeon and specializes in state-of-the-art breast reconstruction.

IMPLANTS

This is the most common type of breast reconstruction— about 75 percent of women get implants. Most of these surgeries involve the use of temporary tissue expanders to stretch the skin and muscles of the chest wall. They are similar to balloons and will be filled with a saltwater solution over time during several office visits. After the skin is adequately stretched, you have a quick surgery for removal of the tissue expanders and placement of permanent implants. You can choose between saline or silicone implants, but most plastic surgeons recommend silicone because they feel more natural. This approach minimizes your recovery and doesn't involve operating on other parts of your body. But implants are man-made things: They may break or cause scar tissue to build up around them (especially if you've had radiation).

Another implant-based reconstruction option takes tissue from the upper back. This is called a latissimus dorsi flap and involves a surgeon moving some latissimus muscle and a small amount of skin and fat from the back to create a breast. Because you usually don't have enough extra tissue on your back, most people also need an implant with this type of surgery.

YOUR OWN TISSUE

Reconstruction can also be done using your own tissue, called autologous reconstruction. The transverse rectus abdominis myocutaneous, or TRAM, flap surgery uses abdominal muscle, skin, and fat to re-create the breast. The good news is you also get a tummy tuck with this reconstruction—a nice little bonus! This is performed two ways: In the first option, called a pedicled TRAM, the blood supply stays attached and the tissue is tunneled under the skin and brought through the mastectomy incision. This surgery can result in a loss of abdominal muscle tone because the surgeon has to cut the rectus muscle, freeing it from the abdomen in order to allow it to move through the tunnel up to the breast. A piece of mesh is then sewn into the lower abdomen to support the area where the muscle was removed. Patients are at risk for hernia formation if this mesh weakens or tears.

The second way to do a TRAM flap is called a free TRAM. Here the abdominal skin, fat, and muscle are completely removed from the body and reattached in the chest using a microscope to connect the blood vessels. Dr. Caterson says this flap has a better blood supply than the standard pedicled TRAM flap, but has the same abdominal weakness problems, as well as a risk for hernia formation.

A state-of-the-art abdominal flap breast reconstruction is another option, called a deep inferior epigastric perforator (DIEP) flap. This procedure can be done only by experienced microsurgeons, and not all plastic surgeons may offer it to their patients. This breast reconstruction also uses the lower abdominal skin and fat, but leaves the rectus muscle behind. Abdominal strength is preserved, and there is no mesh, so there is very little risk of hernia.

Other options include the SGAP, or superior gluteal artery perforator flap. In English, that means building a breast out of the skin and fat of your bum. No muscle is moved. This is sometimes a good option for very thin patients. A second type of buttock flap, called an IGAP, or inferior gluteal artery perforator, flap may also be an option.

Newer options include the transverse upper gracilis, or TUG, flap, which creates a breast out of your inner thigh. Again, only thin patients with extra tissue in this area are good candidates for this procedure.

In general, tissue flap breast reconstructions are pretty extensive procedures with some serious recovery time and recovery pain! However, Dr. Caterson says they give a much more natural-looking result that ages with you, and there is no implant to worry about. Implants may need to be replaced over the course of your (we hope long) lifetime if complications arise.

REALISTIC EXPECTATIONS

You have to be realistic about what you can expect after reconstruction. Many of these procedures leave you with pretty big scars. A naked reconstructed breast does not look like the one God gave you. Most breast reconstruction surgeons will have a photo book you can look at, as well as patients you can call to better understand what to expect.

Sanity Saver

There are wonderful Web sites, such as http://www.breastcancer.org, that have both stories and photos from women who have undergone various procedures. That's a good way to learn about what might work for you. And you can do an Internet search in the privacy of your own home without feeling rushed or uncomfortable about staring at someone else's breasts!

So what if you do have options and have to decide between an implant or your own tissue? Kelley has a friend in Los Angeles with a unique perspective on this issue. Mary Flaherty survived two primary breast cancers thirteen years apart. She is doing just fine. She has lived to see her three children grow up beautifully. Mary had TRAM reconstruction the first time on the right side. When she was diagnosed again with a new cancer on the left side, she elected to have an implant. We asked her to answer some key questions.

Q: **Which side feels and looks more natural?**

A: The more natural-looking reconstruction is the TRAM, although it has the stretch marks on it from the abdominal tissue from my pregnancies. When I went through menopause the first time during chemo, my TRAM breast started getting a little bigger. I asked my doctor about it, and he told me that during menopause women tend to get more abdominal fat and my "breast" is really my abdominal tissue . . . hmmm! This would not happen with an implant! They removed the nipple with the breast so I wound up having to have a tattoo and "button" made on the breast mound. It's not too realistic, but my doctor told me that I would regret not having done the nipple if I was ever in a wet T-shirt contest. (Hasn't happened . . . yet!)

Q: **How did the recoveries differ?**

A: The TRAM recovery definitely took longer, and they did not really have the technique perfected when I had it done in 1997.

    They put me in intensive care so that I could be monitored around the clock, which was not too pleasant. (Fortunately that's not the case anymore. Most women recover on a standard postsurgery floor.)

Q: **Which procedure would you recommend and why?**

A: I would recommend the TRAM procedure since it is your own tissue, feels most natural, and there is not the fear of breakage. I had a sixteen-year-old driver hit me while driving one week after having the implant put in. Luckily in the accident (car airbag vs. breast implant), the implant held up. However, I am always conscious of it potentially breaking when skiing or swimming.

I have also found that my silicone side feels weird at high elevations (we go to Colorado often). Every so often, the implant feels like a foreign object inside of me. It can actually feel cold when the weather is cold. I looked into doing the TRAM a second time but they could not use the same site and I did not want to remove tissue from my thighs or rear end! Plus, I didn't want my right breast to be my stomach and my left breast to be my thigh or butt. Way too confusing!

KELLEY'S RECONSTRUCTION

Kelley ran everything by all her doctors before deciding on a mastectomy with immediate pedicled TRAM reconstruction. At first her radiation oncologist wasn't sure this approach would allow her to give the best, safest radiation, but she was convinced once she saw Kelley's anatomy. Kelley needed both a mastectomy and radiation, so getting all the docs to sign off was essential to moving forward. She really wanted to do everything in one surgery if possible given her responsibilities as a mother with two young children. But obviously the most important thing was getting rid of the cancer effectively and then replacing her breast.

KELLEY: I spent a lot of time before my mastectomy talking to various doctors about reconstruction. It was so confusing. Implants, TRAM, multiple surgeries! I was so overwhelmed that I pretty much talked myself out of reconstruction. I had enough on my plate with the mastectomy, chemo, and radiation. I spoke to one survivor who had a reconstruction horror story and urged me to avoid it all together. But then my wonderful ob-gyn led a growing chorus of friends and family who urged me to spend some time seriously considering reconstruction. I was only thirty-six years old and would hopefully have a long life ahead of me. I was really convinced when a friend's mother who had had a mastectomy twenty years earlier told me she always wished she had a replacement breast all these years. I decided to see a plastic surgeon. He grabbed ahold of my postbaby belly fat and said it would be tight, but he could do the traditional TRAM at the same time as my mastectomy. Sold! All-in-one surgery seemed like the way to go.

I had been warned I would wake up and feel like a Mack truck hit me. Fortunately the pain was not that bad. I was on a lot of medications and had a pain pump attached to my belly. Doctors made an incision around the nipple, which was removed, and took out the breast tissue from that opening. After the plastic surgeon tunneled up from my belly to build the breast, the nipple opening was then covered with belly skin. It definitely looks a bit different.

It was very strange having my stomach sewed so tight that I could not stand up straight for over a week. Ugh. The hardest thing about this surgery was not being able to lift anything for six weeks. I couldn't lift my babies and that was heartbreaking. That also meant I couldn't be alone with them and needed help around the house all the time. TRAM extended my mastectomy recovery period, so I was out of work for a month. That was very difficult. During that time I also had to start chemo. It was a brutal winter for me that year. But I gotta tell you, waking up with a new breast was pretty comforting. It made coping with my mastectomy a lot easier. I said then and I agree now that this was a very good option for me. I have no regrets.

ELISHA'S RECONSTRUCTION

Elisha always knew she would want reconstruction. It became the reward at the end of a long road and a way of putting herself back together. Unfortunately, she was not a candidate for implants because of all the radiation. Her skin would likely not expand enough. She was also very thin with no excess tissue or fat on her stomach for an abdominal flap procedure. This was disappointing news because Elisha had always just assumed that when the time came she would have breast implants and end up with the perfect boobs she'd always admired in other women. Instead, Elisha had to wait two years for her reconstruction. Ultimately her best option was an SGAP (breast from upper bum option), which turned out to be yet another challenging part of her journey.

ELISHA: About halfway through my radiation treatment, I made an appointment to see a plastic surgeon recommended by my breast surgeon. Well, my visit did not go quite as I had planned. After examining me, he told me my best option would be to have latissimus dorsi free flap surgery. It was major surgery and way more complicated than I had expected. The thought of losing muscle in my back scared the you-know-what out of me. I needed someone to tell me there were other options for me. Lesson here, girls, always get a second opinion!

The second surgeon confirmed what I already feared. I had few options available to me. He also felt it was too soon after radiation treatment to get a clear picture of my options. He suggested I come back in six months. In the meantime, my radiation oncologist told me about a fairly new procedure called an SGAP. He said it is an excellent option for women who do not have ample abdominal tissue to donate for breast reconstruction. I did some research and learned that SGAP surgery was a major, eleven-hour surgery, but I thought it might be worth the effort. There are few plastic surgeons trained to perform this procedure——some of the surgeons I consulted didn't even tell me about it. I was fortunate that one of the few surgeons in the country performing this procedure happened to be in Boston. You have to really do your homework to find the best reconstruction options for your unique circumstances.

I planned my surgery around a quiet time in my work schedule. I was calm and at peace going in to have my boob put back on. Almost two years before to the day, I was a basket case having my boob removed! Twelve hours after I was wheeled into the operating room, I woke up in the intensive care unit with a new breast. Those first days after surgery were very painful and uncomfortable. I had three drains in me——two under my arm and one in my butt.

Five days later, I was discharged. I was still shaky and sore, but I was thrilled to be on my way home to recuperate and celebrate my forty-second birthday. But one day into my recovery, I noticed my new breast had turned purple at some point during the night. I knew immediately something was terribly wrong.

We called Dr. Caterson, and she told us to meet her in the emergency room right away. She confirmed that there was a blood clot in my flap. The question now was whether she could save the flap. I immediately underwent five hours of emergency surgery to save my flap. The clot was not a result of anything I did or didn't do. It was most likely a result of the fact that my blood vessels were damaged by all the radiation I'd had, and the blood was not flowing into my new breast as well as it should have. During my second surgery, Dr. Caterson found a big, fat, healthy blood vessel behind my ribs. She had to remove a couple ribs to get at it, but she was able to connect this blood vessel to my SGAP flap. The fact that she was able to save my flap was nothing short of a miracle. Very few flaps have ever been saved from such a compromised situation.

It was a huge scare——for the first time since I had been diagnosed, I actually thought I might die. I had lost a ton of blood and I thought my heart might stop during surgery. I had been under anesthesia for a total of seventeen hours in five days. Doug was so upset and so scared. He had to call our family and friends and try to explain how something that had gone so well had gone so wrong.

I spent the next week in ICU and the following three weeks in the hospital recuperating. I celebrated my forty-second birthday in my hospital room surrounded by tons of flowers and all my dearest family and friends. All that, for a boob! My simple reconstruction turned out to be the hardest part of my cancer experience, but in the end I swear it was all worth it. And keep in mind that my complicated experience was unusual, not what most women can expect!

Now that I have had some time to reflect on the experience, I am still amazed every day how successful my procedure was and how great I look! Still, to this day, I am very careful with my reconstructed breast. For a long time, I was afraid it would fall off. Dr. Caterson told me not to be silly. It is now a part of my body, just like my arms and legs.

Reconstruction is like any other part of this journey. You have to be prepared for anything. Many women undergo several surgeries to get the reconstruction right. You may need surgery on the other side to get an even look. FYI: Your insurance should have to cover adjustments to your nondiseased breast. You ultimately want an appearance that is as balanced and natural as possible. And your insurance should pay for doctors to get the look right for you.

You may need a surgery to create a nipple. This is a relatively minor procedure. In Kelley's case it involved outpatient surgery where the plastic surgeon "pinched" the belly skin on her breast to create a nipple. And then you may have to go back for an in-office visit for tattooing to give the nipple and areola color. The mastectomy may leave you with a crater above your breast. Kelley's plastic surgeon filled that indent in with some thigh fat. Yes, Kelley got liposuction for free just for having breast cancer. Not exactly an even trade, but there are such bright spots along the way. We promise!

MAKING ADJUSTMENTS

Living with a reconstructed breast is an adjustment. You will likely lose all sensation in your breast. You get used to it, but it's still strange. Once at a plastic surgeon's appointment, Kelley's toddler daughter grabbed at her reconstructed breast. The doctor and nurse were laughing, and it took a minute before Kelley even knew what was going on. There really is no sensation!

Kelley was always modest in places like gym locker rooms, but her TRAM makes her even more self-conscious. She usually changes in a shower stall or changing room. She mostly doesn't want someone else to be shocked by her hip-to-hip scar and Franken-boob!

PROSTHETICS

We've spent a lot of time talking about reconstruction, because that's the option we decided was best for us. But many women choose or have only prosthetics as an option. Fortunately the variety and quality of breast forms has improved dramatically over the years.

A breast form is a prosthesis worn either inside a special pocketed bra or attached to your body with adhesives. They range from simple foam or fiber-filled inserts to expensive forms designed by computers that can be attached to the chest. Prices range from several dollars for a "falsie" to several hundred dollars for a silicone form to several thousand dollars for a top-of-the-line custom prosthesis.

Your hospital oncology shop may be a good place to start in your search for prosthetic breasts. Many specialty stores sell prosthetic breasts, and they are often run by women who are survivors and very knowledgeable about living with forms. They are also available at stores such as Sears and Nordstrom.

You will want to spend some time with an experienced fitter to try several options and see which works best for you. Bring along a well-fitted top so you can see what looks best. Your doctor or nurse will likely recommend you wait until six weeks after your mastectomy to schedule a fitting. They can also provide you with a prescription for a prosthesis and prosthetic bra.

Options include:

External silicone is a weighted prosthesis designed to look like natural breast tissue. Because it's weighted, you may have an easier time maintaining your posture and balance.

Nonsilicone forms are lightweight and made of foam or fiberfill. These are good options for exercise, swimming, and for use in hot weather.

An attachable breast is a self-adhesive form that is secured to the chest wall with adhesive strips.

Many mastectomy patients will be given a puff form in a camisole to wear after surgery.

If you have a lumpectomy, you can look for enhancers or partial breast forms you can put in a bra to make the surgical breast match the other side. If you have an expander, there are pieces you can wear in a bra that are filled with material you can remove as the expander gets inflated.

You will want to check with your insurance company ahead of time to find out which postmastectomy products are covered. Usually there is coverage for one breast prosthesis per year and two to four mastectomy bras. You will likely need to submit a prescription from your doctor in order to get reimbursed. Though mastectomy bathing suits are usually not covered, you can purchase stylish swimwear with prosthesis pockets at stores such as Lands' End, Nordstrom, and Sears.

Mary Flaherty wore a prosthesis for seven years. She has a lot of funny stories about it flying out during exercise, nearly exploding at high elevations, and swimming away in pools. As we will talk about in later chapters, you have to keep a sense of humor about all of this. Wigs in particular can cause all sorts of havoc. Seriously, do you want to laugh or cry? You decide.

Au Naturel

Many women will choose to do none of the above. You can certainly live postmastectomy life without reconstruction or prosthesis. Elisha had the experience for two years.

ELISHA: I was never a boob girl, you know what I mean? Big boobs were never a priority for me when I looked at myself in the mirror. I was very thin and small-chested all my life. The most important thing to me was looking good in my clothes. For two years, I had to figure out how I was going to balance having only one breast. What kind of bra was I going to wear? How could I wear a tee shirt? How could I wear a sundress? What about a bikini?

I was very put off about wearing a prosthesis—I don't really know why, but in retrospect I think it had to do with the implications of artificial body parts. Don't fight those feelings; just find a way to work around them. No one way is right or wrong, we all have to go with what works for us. For me,

I ended up wearing a padded bra with no underwire. My sweet friend and coworker made a custom prosthesis for me by sewing together a couple of foam shoulder pads that I would wear in the cup of my bra. It was the perfect solution for me.

For a woman who cares what she looks like (and most of us do!), facing life with one breast, or no breasts, has to be one of the most traumatic, invasive, demeaning moments in your life. Granted, I was so grateful to have my life that I was able to somewhat overlook my disfigured, battered body. I became an expert at making myself look balanced in my clothes, but every morning and every night I had to take them off and face my war wounds in the mirror.

I quickly came to terms with my situation and learned what I was comfortable wearing. No tight T-shirts and no bustier dresses. I'm a total fashionista, so the idea that I could no longer wear anything I wanted to made me angry. At this point, I was still constantly asking, "Why me?" If you are still asking yourself that question, get over it, because there is no answer.

Make a decision about what option works best for you and move forward. You don't have to love or even like your new body, but you will be happier if you can learn to accept it.

Don't Lose Your Sanity!

- Recognize that reconstruction is a process, and it will take a while to get the complete result.
- Learn to live with your new body no matter how scarred and changed it may be. You are alive. That is the most important thing.

- Take the time to research your options before deciding. Good surgeons will never be offended if you ask for a second opinion. They should encourage it, as it will help clarify your options for you.
- Realize you do not have to do anything right now. You may have options later.
- Don't get overwhelmed by all these decisions. Take time out to enjoy music, poetry, or beautiful art.

Don't Lose Your Style!

- Be confident about your new look. A good attitude goes a long way.
- Go shopping and figure out what clothes flatter your new figure.
- Ask for help from friends, other survivors, and thoughtful clothing salespeople to help figure out what works for the new you.
- If your cleavage isn't what it used to be, accent something else that's fabulous, such as your legs or eyes.

Chemo

here are few things in life dreaded as much as the thought of having chemotherapy. It is a very scary process to endure. You are perfectly normal to have anxiety about what lies ahead over the next months. Dr. Partridge says she worries about the people who are not nervous about chemotherapy! It will not be easy, but trust us, you can do this. We'll give you some suggestions about minimizing the unpleasant stuff and maximizing your quality of life.

Both of us were still coping with the aftereffects of major surgery when we had to turn our attention to chemotherapy. If you spend a lot of time worrying about nausea, fatigue, and baldness, you will definitely get overwhelmed. Instead, focus your energy on preparing the best you can to get through this, and rest up. You will need your energy. Take this part of treatment one day at a time.

Years ago everyone got the same chemo cocktail; today chemo is targeted to the individual patient's specific needs and for many women chemo will not be the right choice. Your oncologist will come up with a treatment plan specifically to battle the risks of your cancer.

Is Chemotherapy Necessary?

There are several factors that influence the decision about whether or not to receive chemotherapy for breast cancer. You and your oncologist should take into account the specific features of the cancer (breast cancer is a very heterogeneous disease), your underlying health, and your own preferences when considering whether the risks of chemotherapy are worth it in your situation. You may also be offered additional tests on your tumor such as the Oncotype DX to help you and your doctor make this decision. This test is conducted at a lab in California, and it is useful in predicting the risk of recurrence and the potential benefits from chemotherapy in women with hormone receptor–positive, node-negative breast cancer.

Chemo Before or After Surgery?

Some breast cancer patients are offered chemotherapy before surgery. This may be recommended if a tumor is particularly large in the breast or axilla (underarm), making it difficult for the surgeon to get it all out at surgery. Chemotherapy can shrink a woman's tumor down so that it goes from inoperable to operable. In some cases, women and their doctors will choose to do chemo first in an attempt to shrink a larger tumor so a woman can undergo a lumpectomy instead of a mastectomy. Some doctors prefer this approach so they can see on scans if the tumor is responding to chemo and adjust drugs if necessary.

Studies have shown that this approach is as safe as giving chemotherapy after surgery in the long term. It's best to discuss timing with your oncologist so you can both make the best decisions for your case.

Port or IV?

At some point, your doctor or nurse will likely discuss with you whether you need a port. This is a tube that allows chemo to be delivered to your bloodstream—like an IV—but it goes directly to a large vein in your neck or chest. The end is buried under your skin so that the tube can be accessed when you come in for treatment, and it stays in place even when you go home. Neither of us had ports, but we know many women who did.

A port is implanted in your chest by a surgeon. Your nurse will always be able to access your port, so you won't have to endure painful needle sticks to find a good vein. The port is accessed through a nickel-sized area buried superficially in your chest wall, which is connected to a tube that goes directly into your chest or neck vein. It can also be used to draw blood.

The decision whether to use a port can depend on your treatment plan and number of chemotherapy sessions. The quality of your veins will be another consideration. Kelley opted not to get a port but admits that finding a vein became challenging during her extensive chemotherapy. She was using only one arm for chemotherapy as a precaution against lymphedema. After a while, nurses had to warm up Kelley's arm with a hot towel or hot water to assist in locating a vein.

Dr. Partridge tells patients to try on some of their favorite clothes or a bathing suit to help figure out how to get a port placed in a less noticeable spot. The port will leave a scar on your chest, and you may prefer to have it hidden if possible.

Without a port, you will have to get used to being stuck with needles. A lot! When you go to the cancer center for appointments, make sure you begin the day by letting everyone know you are having chemo. That way perhaps they can stick you just once and use the same line for the rest of the day. We learned that lesson the hard way after having a test such as a heart scan in the morning and then getting "stuck" again later for chemo. This is a good example of learning the system and taking charge of your care. You have to look out for you! Each cancer center has different systems, and you will soon learn the ins and outs of your facility.

CHEMO ORIENTATION

When you have that first chemo orientation—likely with a nurse—bring a notebook and take some notes. You'll need them. You may also want to have a support person there for this appointment. There's a lot of ground to cover when you are starting a treatment this serious. You'll also want to ask about the hospital's systems, such as parking, wait times, scheduling, etc. The more information you have, the better you can try to arrange the treatments so you don't lose your sanity.

A chemo treatment day almost always begins with a blood test. Then you have to wait for the results. You will also be weighed and have your blood pressure and temperature checked. You will likely meet with your oncologist. Then you get your chemotherapy. We're sure you've already learned that you have to be patient when you are a patient. That's certainly true on the infusion floor. One patient says you need to get into "airport mode" on infusion days. That means you should bring a friend or loved one, a book or something to do, and be prepared for delays.

Your first trip to the infusion floor can be a frightening glimpse into your future. You will see people who don't look well, and you may worry that you'll look like them soon. There are great efforts taken to make infusion centers as warm and comfortable as possible, but somehow they always seem to emanate an element of fear and sadness. Try to find that reserve of strength and optimism from within you—you will need it now more than ever.

THE RED DEVIL

There's a lot to learn about the infusion process. Although there are several standard chemotherapy "cocktails," many women currently receive four doses of Adriamycin and Cytoxan, or AC as part of their regime. This is the hard stuff that will almost certainly result in hair loss and make you feel queasy if not downright ill. Elisha had dose-dense treatment, meaning she received these drugs every two weeks. Because she was having this intense course, she needed a drug called Neulasta twenty-four hours after every treatment to boost her white blood cell count. This helped prevent infections and allowed her blood counts to bounce back quickly so she could receive the next treatment on time. Kelley, on the other hand, received her AC every three weeks, which was certainly a bit easier to take.

This chemotherapy is delivered intravenously and usually takes several hours. Adriamycin is sometimes called "the red devil" because of its horrible color and difficult side effects. It's so toxic your chemo nurse will have to put on protective gloves and a gown. He or she will then push the drug into your IV or port instead of allowing it to drip in like the other chemo drugs. It can be a pretty stressful infusion. But instead of viewing it as a toxic drug, try to look at the red devil as a magic potion that will save your life.

ELISHA: My first chemo was scheduled for a Wednesday afternoon. I purposely scheduled the treatment for the end of the day so I could work first. I had done my homework, so I knew to bring a snack and plenty of water. I didn't bring any pillows or blankets, although I know some women take comfort in having their favorite things around them——a cozy pair of slippers, for example.

On the bright side, I loved my infusion nurse, Paula. She was just the sweetest thing ever, as were all the nurses on the infusion floor. It is a calling from God what those nurses do. It is amazing to me how kind and loving they are to every patient. And they are so knowledgeable about the drugs and potential side effects. Your chemo nurse will undoubtedly become a source of important information and strength for you during this time.

I was dressed to the nines as always, wearing the latest Sara Campbell creation, high heels, the hottest new bag, and lipstick perfectly in place. I was still me even though I found myself in a place I never expected to be. I was simply interested in getting in and getting out of my treatment sessions. I was determined not to let this illness rob any more of my precious time than it already had. This was a huge inconvenience in my life! I was committed to fighting cancer, but it would not take over my life or compromise my style.

CONTROLLING THE NAUSEA

Your nurses will explain the dizzying array of antinausea drugs you will take. If you are like us and never had a major health problem in the past, this list of drugs will seem overwhelming and perhaps unnecessary. But, oh no, they are very necessary. Take all of your antinausea medications. Please! This is no time to be a martyr. And if the meds don't work and you feel horrible, don't be shy about asking the docs and nurses what else they have. There might be another option that will work better for you.

Nurses suggest you drink a lot of water the day before your treatment. That will help plump up your veins before chemo day and flush out your system. It's good advice. In fact, try upping your water intake throughout chemo. If you are hydrated you will likely feel a lot better. It will also help with one of the nasty effects of some antinausea drugs: constipation.

If you have never had a constipated day in your life, you may now. These drugs have a real drying effect on your system. Your nurse will likely suggest you add a stool softener or a gentle laxative during chemo. Definitely consider taking that advice. You don't need poopy problems on top of everything else. What's one more pill to swallow! If it doesn't work and you get backed up anyway, ask your team for help.

Your chemo nurse will give you an extensive list of the drugs you need to take. This is a good job for a partner or close friend to manage. They can help make sure you take your pills at the right time. Taking these meds is essential to managing the side effects of these powerful cancer-fighting drugs.

Passing the Time

You are possibly going to be sitting on the infusion floor for several hours. Think seriously about how you want to spend that time. Perhaps you and a loved one want to sit quietly together. Maybe you would prefer to read a book to pass the time. It's okay to bring work as a distraction. Maybe a DVD would help? Or bring your best friend and read *People* magazine and gossip mindlessly about celebrities or your other friends!

This is your time, and you have to think about what best will get you through it. Kelley once asked her book club to come for an AC treatment. They ate popcorn and strawberries and barely talked about the book. But time flew, and Kelley barely thought about the sadness of spending a day on the infusion floor.

It sounds trite, but family and friends really are the best medicine. One time the nurse was having trouble finding a vein for one of Kelley's many infusions. Her friends were there and kept talking as if nothing was wrong. If they weren't there, Kelley would have lost it for sure. A few hot towels and a little creativity by the nurse resulted in the discovery of a good vein. All the while, good conversation and TLC took the stress out of what could have been a horrible day.

ELISHA: I had many dear friends and family who wanted to go with me to chemo treatments. I was so appreciative and loved their support, but halfway through treatment I realized I was spending the whole time entertaining them and trying to keep their spirits up. Honestly, I really just wanted the time alone to read and answer e-mails on my BlackBerry. But inevitably I had someone with me for every treatment. I never allowed my parents to accompany me to a chemo treatment. I knew how difficult my diagnosis was on them, and I wanted to protect them from having to witness this process. In retrospect, I didn't have to worry. My parents showed me more strength and support than I could have ever imagined.

COPING WITH THE SIDE EFFECTS

After that first treatment, you may feel horrible or just a little off. Everybody is different. It's similar to how some of us breeze through a pregnancy while others are sick the entire nine months. Either way, you should probably plan on taking it easy those first few days after chemo. You will want to see how your body reacts.

If you are getting a nausea-inducing chemotherapy regimen (most of them are!), eating may become tricky. You may not feel like eating anything, but it's important to keep up your strength. Try bland carbohydrates such as bagels, toast, or crackers to start. Many people find cold things easier to keep down. Think frozen fruit bars or smoothies. Once you find your comfort food, feel free to stick with it. It's all about staying hydrated and well fed the best you can. Many people do well with small, more frequent, meals. Kelley had luck with smooth soups such as purees. She also developed a serious thing for bagels with peanut butter. Just take it slow and easy.

Hillary Wright, MEd, RD, LDN, a nutritionist at Dana-Farber Cancer Institute, tells patients to first be aware of what side effects could happen and then take one day at a time because everyone tolerates chemo differently. People sometimes have expectations based on someone else's experience, but they may not even have been on the same treatment plan (or even had the same cancer).

Wright suggests you continue to eat as well as you can, if you can, but to be flexible and allow for whatever tastes good at the moment if you're not feeling well. Eating during chemo can also be a little like being pregnant—what usually tastes and smells good may be a total turnoff. If you're feeling a little queasy, opt for bland foods with little smell. Generally, cold foods work because they don't have an odor. Wright suggests prioritizing protein foods like low-fat dairy foods, nuts or nut butters, beans, and cold chicken. It's also important to graze on low-fat carbohydrates throughout the day to help keep your blood sugar and energy levels up. And make sure you drink enough fluids. Wright says getting dehydrated will drain your energy and make it hard to do the things that make life seem normal during treatment.

Some patients find ginger an effective weapon in the war against nausea. In fact, a recent study showed taking ginger supplements with antinausea drugs before chemo can reduce nausea by as much as 40 percent. Of course, ask your oncologist before taking any supplements. But he or she should be fine with you drinking ginger tea. You can make your own with grated ginger root and hot water.

Above all, Wright says to follow your clinician's advice when it comes to taking antinausea medications. They work best at keeping nausea at bay, so take them proactively rather than waiting to feel really nauseated before popping a pill. There is no reason to tough out nausea caused by chemo.

It will just affect your ability to enjoy life to whatever degree is possible between treatments.

You may expect to lose weight during treatment, but most women find the opposite is true. Comfort foods aren't always the lowest in calories! And you may be less active during chemotherapy. Doctors and the latest research recommend that you try to exercise through treatment to prevent weight gain, potentially improve your energy, and keep yourself sane. You may want to ask for a referral to see the cancer center's nutritionist or attend a workshop to help you with any eating issues you may be facing.

Elisha loves her coffee and wine. She looks forward to that cup of coffee or two in the morning and can't wait for a glass of wine or two in the evening! It was awful to basically lose taste for most all foods, including coffee and wine. She wanted to drink only fizzy drinks; flat water made her feel nauseous. She had huge cravings for pasta with red sauce, which she was never able to eat again once she recovered. Be careful about the foods you eat while going through treatment. You may never want to see them again afterward because of the strong negative association.

The important thing to remember about chemo is that the effects are often cumulative, especially the fatigue. Ultimately, this part of chemo will likely kick your ass. You may just have one or two bad days following treatment or simply be wiped out. We all respond differently. AC will, at the very least, slow you down a bit. Trust us, this really isn't something to conquer but rather endure. You just want to get through it and get it over with.

As with anything we do in life, attitude and a positive mindset can help get you through each difficult day. As much as you may want to, you cannot walk away from this situation. You have to stay and fight the fight, so you might as well embrace it and make it the best experience possible. The sooner you let go of any "Why me?" anger the more tolerable this treatment will be for you and those around you.

That said, Kelley can distinctly remember mourning the loss of her good health. It is no fun to be a patient when you used to be healthy. Kelley had a mini breakdown a week after her first treatment and just cried. She had spent a lot of that week at home feeling lousy and missing her regular routine. Crying did make her feel better, and then she went back home where the kids usually did a good job of cheering her up. The routine of her young family's life proved to be a great distraction from the stress of treatment.

You may find yourself getting increasingly run down. At some point you may have problems with your blood counts. These treatments wipe out a lot of good cells along with the bad ones. There can also be serious complications, such as infections, that can occur during chemotherapy. You may start to feel like a bit of a zombie. You will go places and feel like you're there but not really engaged in what's going on around you. It's not fun to lose your pep and energy. You will hear the expression "chemo brain." It refers to the experience some patients have with loss of concentration and memory during and after treatment. You'll go to say something and can't get the words out. Or you'll start a sentence and forget where you were going with that thought. It is very frustrating.

KELLEY: Toward the end of my AC treatments, I caught a cold from my kids. When is a cold not just a cold? When you have cancer and are getting chemotherapy! Although I probably had the same bug, likely viral, as my kids, the fever I spiked raised alarms with Dr. Partridge. She explained that even though it may be just a cold, a fever during chemotherapy could also be a sign of a more serious infection. So over Easter weekend I found myself in the emergency room getting all sorts of tests, including blood counts and chest X-rays, to make sure nothing serious was going on. It was a low point in my treatment and a very frightening experience for those around me. The wonderful ER team gave me IV fluids to hydrate me, and I started to perk up again. Everything turned out okay, but it shows how concerned doctors can become when they have given you drugs that can make your blood counts go low. That weekend was one of my lowest points in a year of some pretty tough moments.

MOUTH SORES

You may find yourself with mouth issues such as canker sores, an annoying potential side effect from these drugs. You can try over-the-counter drugstore remedies or simple rinses with salt and warm water. They are truly a pain. If they are really bad, especially if you are having trouble eating, your doctor may prescribe a numbing mouthwash or pain medication.

YOUR SENSES

You may develop a slightly metallic taste in your mouth, and your sense of smell may become heightened and sensitive. *Good Morning America*'s Robin Roberts shared on air how Diane Sawyer's perfume would make her feel sick. Needless to say, Diane kindly refrained from wearing perfume for a while. You may just have a constant queasy feeling for a while. For some, it is like being pregnant and just feeling off.

And, sadly, you may lose your sense of taste. This is a truly cruel side effect. You may finally feel well enough to eat your favorite food only to find you can no longer taste it! It's the strangest feeling to take a bite of something wonderful and discover it has no taste at all. Fortunately all of these side effects will likely go away once you finish treatment.

Complementary Therapies

So what are you going to do about these side effects? We strongly recommend you look into complementary therapies. They can lift your spirits and help ease side effects. The great news is that many cancer centers now offer these services on-site, and more doctors understand how they can benefit their patients. Kelley had acupuncture a few days before her AC treatments to help with nausea. She would also try to go to a yoga class before getting her infusions. It calmed her anxious mind and helped her relax. Reiki can be very powerful as well, and massage has proven benefits that you may want to explore. Just make sure to clear any complementary therapy with your oncologist first and be up-front with providers about your situation. Your oncologist will also want to know about any supplements you might take, as there can be potential interactions with treatment.

Get Moving

We strongly encourage you to get up and exercise. Neither of us liked to exercise all that much prior to diagnosis. But we were so frightened by our diagnosis we decided we had to stay one step ahead of the Grim Reaper! Oh, c'mon, you can't lose your hair and your sense of humor. We're just kidding.

But you do need to keep moving. We recommend exercising and laughing at the same time whenever possible. Go for a walk with a friend and keep the mood light. Talk about anything other than cancer. Try exercising at a gym or at home and watching something like *The Ellen DeGeneres Show*. Guaranteed you will find yourself laughing even if you're bald, nauseous, and have one boob. Seriously. Kelley would also bring sneakers to the cancer center and take a walk between appointments. She would do anything to get out of the sterile hospital environment and breathe fresh air.

If you can, plan a short getaway during your chemo treatments.
Take a day trip or a weekend away to lift your spirits. Go visit a
friend who can offer you encouragement. This part of treatment can
be so draining, and you may need a lift to keep you going. If you can
get away, your spirit will be stronger!

ELISHA: I remember right before my last chemo treatment my dear friend took a trip with me to Palm Beach for a little R&R. We stayed at our friend's home right on the ocean. We spent time walking on the beach and reading by the pool. One afternoon while we were sitting by the pool, Ginger took a picture of me—I was wearing a leopard bikini with one boob and a bald head. It's a fabulous picture, and I keep it on my desk in my office because I never want to forget what I went through to save my life. I also love the fact that I never compromised my style even though my body had changed so dramatically.

TAXANE DRUGS

After or during AC, or instead of an AC-type of regime, you may be treated with a taxane chemotherapy, either as a single agent or in combination. Your exact treatment plan will depend on your unique situation. Elisha and Kelley both received twelve weekly treatments of Taxol following AC. You may get a taxane drug combined with Herceptin if you are HER2/neu positive or the drug Taxotere, often paired with Cytoxan (instead of AC), in a regimen called TC.

Your wonderful chemo nurses will take steps to make sure you don't have a bad reaction to these drugs. That means you will have an infusion of what's called "premeds" first. Often the first infusion of a taxane drug is a long, slow process as the nurses try to gauge how your body is responding to the treatment.

The premeds can include Zantac and Benadryl, which can make you feel very sleepy. Kelley dropped an entire smoothie all over herself and a friend coming out of treatment one night. She literally felt drunk! Don't make any plans after these infusions and, for goodness' sake, don't drive yourself home. You will probably head straight to bed. You may want to ask your doctor if you can slowly reduce or cancel the premeds if you are not having any adverse reactions. Steroids may also be given to prevent a reaction with the taxane drugs. Some patients have reported breaking out with pimples and having trouble sleeping at night after treatment.

People may tell you the taxane drugs are much easier to take than AC, but you may just have different problems. Some people suffer from muscle, bone, and joint aches. They can be treated with ibuprofen and Tylenol and will go away. The fatigue may continue to be a major challenge. If you still have eyebrows and eyelashes, they may fall out. Your finger- and toenails may turn strange colors and/or fall off. You may have already been struggling to have some healthy-looking color in your face. These taxane drugs may turn you a shade of gray. It's no fun. You may find yourself coping with neuropathy. This is a tingling in your fingers and toes that may not go away until after treatment ends. Kelley still struggles with occasional neuropathy in her feet and toes. It's a very annoying side effect. No doubt about it, this part of the slog gets hard. And you are still at risk for blood counts going low with all these regimes, which may result in anemia, fever, or infection.

Considering Clinical Trials

One of your doctors may suggest you are a good candidate for a clinical trial, or you may see a sign-up at one of your provider's offices. Kenneth Getz is the founder of the Center for Information and Study on Clinical

Research Participation (CISCRP). We asked him to explain a little bit about what you need to know about clinical trials.

Q: How can a breast cancer patient find appropriate clinical trials?

A: Studies are regularly advertised in newspapers and on the radio and TV. They're posted on bulletin boards in cancer centers and in physician waiting rooms. You can proactively turn to a number of sources for information as well. Among the most trusted sources are your primary care and specialty-care physicians and nurses. Local and national breast cancer support and advocacy groups may be excellent sources of information. There's also a great deal of information available on the Internet: The National Library of Medicine maintains the most comprehensive listing of breast cancer clinical trials funded by government agencies, foundations, and industry. This listing can be found at http://www.clinicaltrials.gov. Another, less comprehensive, listing of breast cancer clinical trials funded by industry can be accessed at http://www.centerwatch.com.

Q: What should a patient consider before enrolling in a trial?

A: Before volunteering for any clinical trial, there are two essential questions that you need to ask first: "Do I have all of the information that I need to make an informed choice?" and "How far am I willing to go?" For patients and their families facing a serious, life-threatening illness, these questions are often easy to answer. But for less severe though unpleasant illnesses, these questions may be more difficult to answer. Gathering all the information that you need to make an educated decision will take some time. As we say at CISCRP, education must come before participation. In my book, *The Gift of Participation,* I list hundreds of questions and areas that you'll need to consider. Here's a sampling:

ABOUT THE CLINICAL TRIAL

What is the main purpose of the study?

What are the chances that this drug will work?

How long will the clinical trial last?

What kinds of risks are involved?

How much of my time will the study take?

What are my chances of getting a placebo?

What kind of adverse reactions or side effects have other people (or animals) experienced?

ABOUT YOUR COMPENSATION AND COSTS

Do I have to pay for any part of the study? If so, will insurance cover these costs?

Do I have to talk to my health insurance company before enrolling in the study?

Will I be paid for my participation?

Q: What are the risks and benefits of participating in a clinical trial?

A: There are numerous risks and benefits. It is critically important that patients weigh all of the risks and benefits in order to determine whether a clinical trial is right for them. You should discuss these risks and benefits with your family and your physician or nurse.

Among the most common benefits include the opportunity to gain access to experimental new treatments and expert medical attention. Participants receive free treatment and medical procedures associated with the clinical trial. Many volunteers consider the impact that their participation will have on advancing medical knowledge and ultimately helping patients—including family members—in the future a major benefit.

There are many risks: Participants may experience serious adverse reactions to the study medication. The treatment they receive during the clinical trial may not be effective. Typically in breast cancer clinical trials, patients will not receive a placebo, but they may receive a standard or already approved treatment instead of the experimental study drug. Many clinical trials require a lot of visits, and many include blood and lab work and even some invasive and unpleasant procedures that present some risk to the patient.

At CISCRP, we frequently say that behind every medicine and treatment are people who gave the gift of participation in clinical trials. Without people to volunteer for clinical trials, the world would be a far different place. New diseases would flourish. Well-known diseases—many of which are managed today with medication and lifestyle changes—would instead cripple, disfigure, or kill. Without such drugs as Herceptin, tamoxifen, and Gleevec, many adults and children stricken with cancer would be buried or facing the end of life as opposed to fighting the disease and living longer productive lives.

Participating in clinical trials is an entirely personal decision. We are both participating in ongoing written surveys and a tumor sample study about young women that Dr. Partridge is conducting. Its goal is to figure out more about the unique characteristics and effects of breast cancer in young women. This required very little time or effort and no risk. Kelley also participated in an exercise study during cancer treatment. It involved submitting weekly reports detailing exercise during chemotherapy. It actually was a huge benefit to Kelley because it inspired her to keep moving!

You have to decide whether a clinical trial is right for you. Though some have more risk, most have potential benefits. A patient's small role in a clinical trial can often lead to big discoveries down the road.

Having a Life

It may feel like chemotherapy is sucking the life out of you in order to save you. But you can still have a life. Kelley took a leave from work after her surgery but did go back on a reduced schedule during chemotherapy. She would usually go into the television station for three or four days most weeks and tried to take on less challenging assignments. (No racing around at fire or murder scenes!) Elisha missed only one or two days of work during treatment. She organized her travel schedule around her "up" weeks. Despite the rigors of chemo, she put together fashion shows, took care of Doug, spent time with loved ones, and raised money for breast cancer research. Staying busy helped us both keep our minds off the fears and challenges of our fight. Kelley continued to care for her children and found they kept her laughing even when she felt horrible. You know your body and what your responsibilities entail. Don't try to be a hero, but don't give into the cancer too much, either. Find a balance that works for you given your unique situation.

Kelley thought of this whole ordeal at times as a boxing match. Long regimes of chemotherapy will undoubtedly make you feel like you are pinned to the ropes or on the floor. It is tough to keep taking the hits and going back for another round each week.

KELLEY: When I looked at the daunting schedule of twelve weekly Taxol and Herceptin treatments, after I had finished AC, I knew I had to do something to help myself through this. I immediately sent out an e-mail to my amazing extended family and closest friends and rallied the troops. I really hadn't directly asked for help until then. I sat back and let others coordinate for me. This time I asked for the amazing women in my life to sign up for a spot and come keep me company. (Brendan came one week, too, but not every week! I wanted him to work and have that escape from the cancer.) Each week I looked forward to the company of a new loved one. Those were special Mondays. It was great to have three uninterrupted hours of conversation with another adult. It was actually heaven for a mom of young kids. I now know how most of my friends met their husbands. I got to pal around with my mom and sisters like we used to do when we lived under one roof. We shared an intimate experience that has deepened my family relationships and my friendships. It is one of the gifts cancer gave me. Truly it is.

Later, when Kelley switched to an every-third-week schedule of Herceptin treatments, she was mostly on her own. Dana-Farber had weekend appointments for infusions without a doctor's appointment, so Kelley would often just run in by herself on a Sunday and bring the newspaper for company. Chemo had gotten pretty routine at that point. It was just easier to go in and get it over with on a weekend day.

ELISHA: I walked into the infusion room every other Wednesday with a sunny attitude, as if I was going to a cocktail party. I was happy and upbeat and usually looking forward to whatever plans I had made with friends after my treatment. This positive attitude spread like wildfire with my fellow patients in the infusion room. The nurses in the hospital told me I was an inspiration to all the other patients around me. One woman who was on the same chemo schedule told me she was feeling so hopeless and unattractive, and I inspired her to put on lipstick, get dressed, and move on with her treatment. This was the most amazing compliment I've ever received.

Don't Lose Your Sanity!

- Use your chemo time the way you want.

- Speak up if the antinausea drugs aren't working or if any other symptoms are getting you down. Don't be a martyr.

- Take it one day at a time. Don't get overwhelmed by fear of the unknown.

- Smile, especially when you are on the infusion floor.

- Do what you want when you can. Ask for help when you cannot continue your work and home routine.

Don't Lose Your Style!

- You can be stylish and comfortable while having your chemo treatment.

- A smile and a positive attitude are the hottest accessories you can own.

- Keep your sunscreen handy at all times. Some chemo drugs make you susceptible to sunburns. Avoid exposure when possible.

- If you can, make time to pamper yourself. Plan a short getaway or make a spa appointment—anything to take your mind off the stress of chemo.

Hair Today, Gone Tomorrow

if you need chemotherapy, then you may be about to lose your hair. That means everywhere. Sorry to say, ladies, but you could soon look like a bald eleven-year-old. If you have no boobs, you'll look like an eleven-year-old boy. The good news: You may not need a bikini wax anytime soon!

Or you could be like some of Dr. Partridge's patients. They tell her they lost hair in the places they wanted to keep it and kept hair they wanted to lose! Ugh.

We cannot lie to you. This sucks. Losing our hair was one of the saddest experiences of our lives. And the buildup can be very stressful.

Kelley was about to lose her hair and had her three-year-old's birthday party and goddaughter's christening to attend. All she wanted was her hair to stay put for those events. It did. You learn to cherish small victories over this disease. But days later, her hair was gone.

No matter how prepared you think you are to lose your hair, when it actually happens it is terrifying. It is a total shock to see your bald self in the mirror, and it makes you feel and look like a cancer patient. The good news is that it's only hair and it will eventually grow back. The trick is to figure out how to look your best while feeling your worst.

Preparing for Hair Loss

The general rule of thumb is you will start to lose your hair ten to fourteen days after your first standard chemotherapy treatment. We suggest you cut your hair short well before that in preparation. It may be easier to cope with this dramatic change if you do it in stages. If you want to wear a wig, it's best to go out shopping before your hair falls out, so you can find a wig that best re-creates your precancer look.

Then you have to decide what to do about your impending hair loss. You may start to feel a little tingling or discomfort before your hair goes. Then you will notice hair loss when you brush or run your fingers through your mane. You can wait at this point for it all to go. But you need to keep in mind, you may wake up with a lot of hair on the pillow. You may be scooping up clumps of hair in the shower. It's not pretty.

ELISHA: To say that I was the vainest hair person ever would be an understatement! I had been a cash cow to my hairdresser for many years with my regular weekly blowouts. I took great pride in my long, blond flip and, like most women, my hair had become a part of my identity. The thought of losing it was very upsetting. Still, I decided to take the bull by the horns, and two weeks before I started chemo, I had it all cut off. The shorter it was, the less traumatic it would be when it all started to fall out. I did not want to face long, blond clumps of hair on my pillow in the morning or in my shower drain. The hair had to go, and a new fashion statement was about to begin.

Buzz Cut

Another option is to shave it all off once it starts to go. This sounds radical and scary, and in some ways it is. But you may find it's the most empowering way to handle a situation over which you have no control.

You can ask your partner to do the shaving. You can ask your hair stylist to do it in a private area. You probably want to cut off as much hair as possible and then use an electric razor. You can include your kids in this process if you think they can handle it. Even if you are able to keep a sense of humor with friends and family around, there may be a very serious letdown afterward.

KELLEY: My hair started falling out about two weeks after my first chemo treatment. A strand here, a strand there. I started to avoid washing or even brushing my hair. For me, I knew it was time to shave my head after baby Cecilia grabbed my hair and got a fistful. Madeline complained at dinner she had a hair on her plate. It was totally gross, and I was done.

My sister Melissa and my best friend, Liz, came for support as my hairdresser shaved it all off. Once he had cut off most of my hair, he started to shave it. Suddenly I looked badass. I had transformed from the girl next door to a rock star. I felt tough. I wanted to beg someone to mess with me. I had been stripped down once again by this disease, but I was surprised by what a tough layer we found underneath my TV bob. I paraded around the newsroom emboldened by the new me.

I wish I could say that feeling lasted all week long. Instead, I found myself feeling a little less rock star each day. I think of myself as having a lot of self-confidence, but this hair thing instantly makes you look like a cancer patient. I didn't look sick or feel like a patient until my hair was gone. Suddenly I found myself totally self-conscious. Should I wear the wig? Too obvious. Bandana? Okay for the gym. A hat? What if it blows off? I just didn't feel comfortable with any of my options. None felt like me.

Kelley did donate her hair to charity, and that's something you may want to consider. She picked Locks of Love (http://www.locksoflove.org), an organization that provides wigs for children with hair loss. Your hair is supposed to be at least ten inches long, but if it's short they will often still take the donation and sell it to offset costs. The Pantene Beautiful Lengths program (http://www.beautifullengths.com) requires only eight inches of hair. It donates free wigs to women across the country. Donating your hair is one way to turn a negative into a positive.

Wigs

Given Kelley's on-air television job she decided to go with a high-quality wig. She was also trying to maintain a sense of normalcy for her kids and found she did not like people's reactions when she looked like a cancer patient. One day Kelley decided to walk her kids to school wearing a pink bandana. All across Boston she got pathetic looks from everyone who saw her walking a double stroller with the very obvious bandana on. Kelley wanted to crawl into a shell. She just couldn't stand other people's pity. That day she wasn't feeling pathetic at all!

To find the right wig, Kelley went into a salon before her hair fell out and tried on a bunch of wigs. She was able to see the difference between wigs. The prices were a big consideration. Most of us have no idea how expensive wigs can be.

Sanity Saver

Check with your insurance company before you go wig shopping to find out how much they will cover. Then you need to get your doctor or nurse to write you a prescription that you will need to submit for reimbursement. It's helpful to know as early as possible how much your insurer will cover. In some states a wig is also tax free because it is a medical prosthesis.

After picking out your wig, you might want to have your hairdresser cut and style it to match your existing 'do. That's how you get the most natural look.

Nikki Walsh is the president of PK Walsh, which has been helping women with hair loss issues in the Boston area for twenty-five years.

Q: How do you pick out a wig?

A: As soon as you know you will need one you will want to start looking. It helps to bring a close friend who will give honest feedback, as this can be a terrifying experience. Nurses can usually recommend places to find a wig based on what they have seen and liked in other patients. Have a consultation before you lose your hair. It's important that the consultant you meet with has a good idea of how your hair looks. If you have a favorite picture, bring it along. Also, the salon you choose should be easily accessible for you. That's because you will need a few visits before you are finished with your purchase.

Q: How much can a patient expect to spend and why are wigs so expensive?

A: Cost can vary from salon to salon. Insurance typically will pick up a portion of the wig. For a high-quality wig, prices can range from $250 to thousands of dollars. When shopping around for the best place to buy your wig, make sure they have a private fitting room. The last thing you want is to take your hair off in the front of a salon. And make sure stylists know how to size and cut. Some salons may be able to sell you the wig but provide little or no follow-up. Once you lose your hair, the wig fits differently and you will need custom sizing. Try to find a salon that specializes in hair loss. You do not want to have a bad experience or work with someone who does not know enough to help.

Q: Do you have to spend a lot of money to get a great-looking wig?

A: It depends on what your own hair looks like and if you have a preference for the type of hair you choose. Hair is available in synthetic; blend, which is half synthetic and half human hair; and human hair. Comfort is more important than style or color. If it is a good or higher quality wig, it will look less "wiggy." How you wear it makes a difference as well. It is crucial to hide any perimeters of the wigs if they show. Some of the nicer wigs will allow you to not wear bangs or have a very natural-looking hair line. Get what you feel comfortable and confident in. If you feel good about the way you look, everyone around you will feel good.

You can bring the wig back to the salon every few weeks to have it cleaned and styled or you can ask stylists to teach you how to do it yourself. Some of the salons specializing in wigs provide cut, shape, combs, and lessons as part of the purchase. You may also want to experiment with wig caps to see if they help you get a good fit. Those are tight head coverings that you wear over your head and under your wig.

Kelley ended up with two wigs and would rotate them. One was a durable everyday look, and the other was a longer, more elegant wig. She actually never styled them herself, preferring to let her hairdresser wash and blow them out every two weeks. Honestly, one benefit is that your hair always looks good. And wearing a wig is a huge timesaver in the morning. You just put it on and go. Kelley is very active and never had many wig mishaps. They actually stay on pretty well if you get a good fit.

For the gym, beach, and more casual outings, Kelley found an amazing product that worked well for her. It's called Hat & Hair (http://www.hatandhair.com). It's a piece of hair that you can attach inside any hat or baseball cap with Velcro. It's not perfect, and anyone who studied you probably could tell something was a bit off. But it really worked well for weekends and the gym. That's how Kelley also solved the challenge of swimming. Kelley found Hat & Hair products at her cancer center's oncology shop.

Remember how Elisha mentioned that long, blond flip she used to care so much about? Now she wears a short, chic style. It's a look she developed during treatment and now embraces.

ELISHA: I knew I would never wear a wig. I don't say this as a criticism; clearly there is nothing wrong with wearing a wig. It just was not for me. I felt there was something sneaky about it. I know that sounds crazy, but I never tried to hide the fact that I had breast cancer. I was not ashamed of it, and it definitely was not my fault. You know the saying "bald is beautiful"? Well I adopted that mind-set and got on with my life. One of my colleagues in

New York City said to me, "You are the chicest bald woman ever." Plus, I had Hermes scarves that I had been collecting all my life, so I decided to put them to good use.

It just so happened that my treatment occurred during the winter months in the Northeast, which can be very cold. During the day I was fine wearing a scarf or a hat, but at night in bed my head would get cold. No one warned me how sensitive a bald head can be. I ended up going to the boutique in my hospital and buying a little cotton cap like a baby would wear. I wore it to bed every night, and it kept my head warm and protected. I would also massage a little extra virgin olive oil into my scalp before putting on my cotton cap. I definitely was not creating any new fashion trends with this look, but it really helped to keep my scalp from getting dry and cracked.

How to Tie a Scarf

To get a great look with a scarf, fold it in half, corner to corner. Place the scarf over your head with the corners facing out. Wrap the right and left corners around the back and tie them at the nape of your neck.

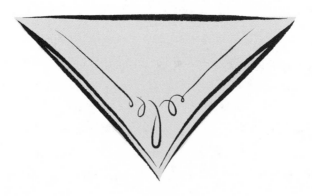

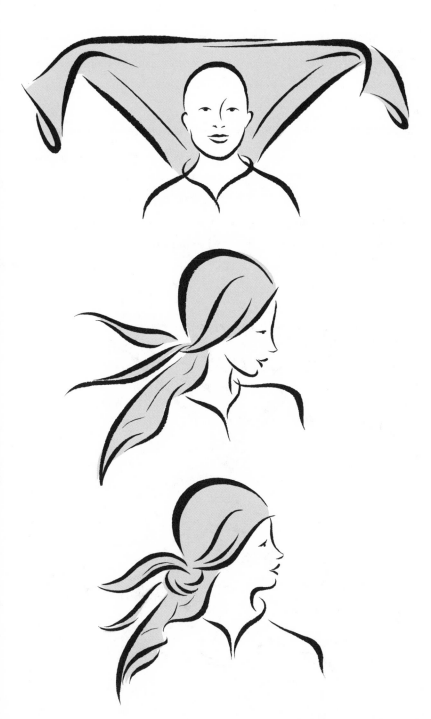

ANOTHER GREAT SCARF OPTION

Fold a square scarf in a triangle, corner to corner, then take the bottom corner and fold it back into the center. Place the scarf centered on your head. Take the sides and wrap them around the back of your head and back around to the center top of your head. You can tie it in a bow or a knot on top of your head. For a dressier look, tie it in a knot and pin a brooch in the knot. It gives you the look of an elegant turban.

You can also go around bald if you choose. If you are okay with your look, why worry about other people's reactions? That's their problem. But they *will* have reactions, and that may be your problem! So think carefully about what you want to do now. You can always try out different options until you find one that works for you.

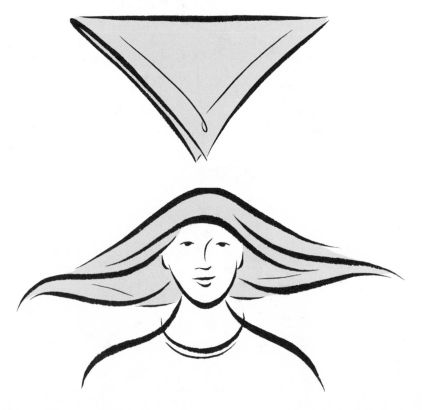

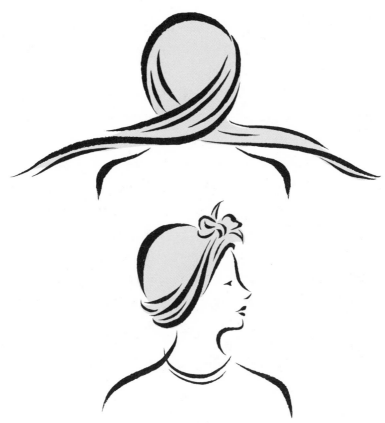

The New You

It will take a while to get back to looking like you. You might experience something called "chemo curls," the all-too-common experience of even straight hair coming back in curly. It can be a bit strange to deal with if you were used to straight hair. You can experiment with flat irons to see if you can set your hair straight again. There are mini flat irons available that may work well with cropped, curly locks. Try experimenting with straightening shampoos and conditioners. Hair waxes can be effective at taming a curly mane. Be patient; your original hair texture will return in time. Hair can also change color, either temporarily or permanently. Dr. Partridge says it's okay to start coloring your hair again when and if you want to.

You will also have to decide at some point when to stop covering up your head. There's an awkward time when the wig just won't fit right anymore, but your hair may not be long enough for you to be comfortable without it. Kelley shaved her head in March of that horrible year and by the end of December she was ready to face the world with her new cropped 'do. But there were a lot of bad hair days to contend with over the following few months. It can be really hard to manage the hair as it comes in and try to look good. To be honest, it was almost another year after that until Kelley had a look that felt like her again. The good news is that Kelley's hair grew in thicker than it was before, and is actually quite nice. Getting comfortable with the new you is a process. Most of us liked the way we looked before cancer!

Throughout this hairless period, try to keep your sense of humor. Mishaps will happen. You may get strange or sad looks that make you angry. You may find the kids in your life are fascinated with your baldness. Kelley's young nieces and nephews always asked to see the wig or her bald head.

KELLEY: We were sitting outside having lunch on Martha's Vineyard with my parents and the kids. Midmeal my then three-year-old Maddie reached over and yanked off my wig. I was sitting there on a porch full of diners with a bald head. My mother's jaw just dropped. She was stunned. I just put the wig back on and kept eating as if nothing happened. Who gives a crap? I didn't know any of those people. And I didn't want to yell at Maddie because anyone with kids knows she would just do it again if I made a big deal out of it! I had survived wind, rain, and snow with my wig intact. But I was no match for a three-year-old. Can't lose your wig *and* your sense of humor, right?

Don't Lose Your Sanity!

- Remember, this too shall pass!
- Your hair will come back and may be better than ever.
- Ask those closest to you to tell you honestly what looks best.
- If you want, ignore the critics! Go with what makes you feel comfortable.
- You are still your fabulous self with or without hair.

Don't Lose Your Style!

- Experiment with what works best for you.
- Get a new short haircut before your hair starts to fall out.
- Take the time to find a wig that makes you feel comfortable.
- Spend time with your hair stylist to make your wig look as close to your own hair as possible.
- Your leg and arm hairs may come back ingrown. Products such as Tend Skin may help if you are having a lot of ingrown hairs.
- Wear color! Wearing clothes in bright, happy colors always makes you look and feel better.

SEVEN

Radiation, aka "Groundhog Day"

the good news is that radiation does not hurt, and its side effects are usually tolerable and temporary. The bad news is that this treatment can present yet another mental challenge.

By the time you have survived surgery and perhaps completed your chemotherapy treatment, you might feel like you can take on any challenge. You're right! Radiation therapy is not a cakewalk, but after chemo you will likely find it much easier physically. But make no mistake: It is an extremely important part of the mission to save your life.

Radiation therapy is one of the most common treatments for many different types of cancer. Many people become cancer free after receiving radiation treatment alone or in combination with surgery or chemotherapy. Unlike chemo, which exposes your entire body to cancer-fighting chemicals, radiation focuses only on the site where the tumor was and the surrounding area.

A Commitment of Time and Energy

Fighting cancer is a huge commitment of time and energy, and radiation is no exception. For patients, it's not too much fun to go to the hospital every day for six weeks. It gets old fast.

But such a long course of treatment is traditionally recommended because it increases the chances that the radiation will hit cancer cells when they're growing. Spreading out treatments is also the best way to protect your healthy cells, because each dose of radiation is relatively small.

We both did our best to keep a good attitude during our six-week slog through radiation. We weren't happy about the inconvenience breast cancer had become in our lives. We wanted to live, so we did what we were told. But we certainly hadn't put our lives on hold so far and we weren't willing to do so now. Once again we tried to balance some sort of normal routine with yet another time-consuming treatment.

You will probably get the traditional course of radiation, but there's a chance you'll be on different plans. They include:

Accelerated breast irradiation: Some doctors are now giving slightly larger daily doses over only about three weeks. In some cancer centers, patients are getting even larger doses of radiation to part of the breast in just five days.

Intraoperative radiation therapy (IORT): In this approach, a single large dose of radiation is given in the operating room right after lumpectomy before the breast incision is closed.

Kelley's radiation oncologist was Dr. Julia Wong at Dana-Faber Cancer Institute in Boston. We asked her to answer some key radiation questions.

Q: Why is radiation traditionally six weeks long?

A: We have an established range of total doses that, when given in a small dose per day for a number of weeks, will give the best likelihood of being effective at eliminating microscopic disease and yet have a reasonably low chance of causing both long-term and short-term side effects. In patients who have had a lumpectomy, this often consists of whole breast radiation for four and a half to five weeks, followed by a "boost"— continued radiation directed just toward a smaller area around the tumor site.

Q: Why are some women getting shorter courses of treatment?

A: There is evidence from a group in Canada and other institutions that giving slightly higher doses per day, and doing fewer treatments in selected patients, yields similar results when compared to "standard" whole breast radiation, both in terms of side effects and efficacy.

Q: Is there a magic cream or other way to prevent burns?

A: No. My experience has been that skin reactions are highly individual, not predictable based on history of reaction to sun or baseline sensitivity, and are not preventable with topical preparations. Sometimes we need or want to cause a skin reaction, depending on the cancer situation. This is usually in the postmastectomy setting, in which the radiation is being directed at the skin of the chest wall in addition to the underlying tissue and possibly lymph node. So, in those settings, a burn of sorts is actually desirable, from the physician's perspective anyway.

PREPARING FOR RADIATION

You will begin this part of treatment by meeting with your radiation oncologist and/or a nurse. They will lay out what to expect in terms of the treatment and go over the logistics. You can expect to learn what the radiation will do and how you can best care for your skin.

Radiation essentially is designed to kill cancer cells and shrink tumors. It will damage both cancer cells and normal ones, but most normal cells can bounce back and function properly again.

To best target the bad guys, you will need very precise treatment. That's why you will go for something called radiation "mapping," or simulation. This will likely take a few hours and will be done in the hospital or cancer center. The doctors will use images, sometimes made with a special CT scanner, and make precise measurements. You may feel like a science experiment lying on that table having everyone examining you. Lying on your back with your arms over your head is not the most comfortable position. But it's essential that the mapping be done as accurately as possible so you get the correct dose of radiation in the right places. Your radiation oncologist is also working hard to keep the radiation away from your essential organs, such as your lungs and heart. This is serious stuff.

KELLEY: I was an emotional mess on my mapping day. I had just endured six months of chemotherapy, and I was spent. When I arrived for my mapping and got up on that table, I was a basket case. I just felt so exposed and vulnerable lying there, arms up over my head while everyone worked around my chest. I felt overwhelmed thinking about taking on another six weeks of treatment. My emotional reserves were nonexistent. I started to cry. I found myself getting increasingly fed up with being a patient. Everyone was so nice, but I had just had it!

TATTOOS

At this session you will also get your radiation tattoos. They are very small dots that allow the radiation therapists to line you up properly in the machines each day. Again, it's very important that these markings are done precisely. It doesn't really hurt—just a pinch for a second or so.

Still, you may find these tattoos annoying. Frankly, we don't mind them so much. They are rather small and rarely can be seen when you're wearing clothes. If you prefer low-cut styles, you can always look into laser tattoo removal, but you may want to check with your radiation oncologist before doing anything to those marks. Dr. Wong says she doesn't encourage removal as a precaution in case you ever need radiation in the future and are trying to avoid treating the same area again. A safe compromise may be to remove the upper, most visible, tattoo but keep the others in place. This is another decision you need to think through carefully and discuss with your radiation oncologist. Each doctor may have a different take on this issue. But that's something to worry about down the road. For now you just need to think about getting through the next six weeks.

GETTING STARTED

At your orientation, you may be warned that lotions, powders, deodorants, and antiperspirants can interfere with radiation, so you may be advised not to use them during treatment. You may be told not to shave your armpit on the affected side, and you may receive a list of vitamins to avoid because they can interfere with radiation. Dr. Wong says a multivitamin is usually okay, but she prefers patients avoid large doses of antioxidants that could interfere with treatment.

At this session, you may be able to talk to the nurse about radiation schedules. Often, though, you cannot get a slot until just before your treatment begins. The morning slots are usually the most popular and hardest to get. Keep in mind that you may be able to start in one time slot and move once someone else finishes treatment.

Radiation itself is not painful. You will get used to a routine of changing, waiting, and then heading into the machine. You will lie on your back with your arms over your head. The radiation will likely take only a few minutes. Once the therapists have you in the correct position, they will leave the room. Usually they can still see you through a window or a monitor. They are right there should you have any concerns or questions. You will know you are getting the radiation because of the whirring noises of the machines. You'll get to know them by heart. But you won't actually feel the radiation.

You'll want to stay very still so the radiation beams hit the right spots. You can breathe, though. Try taking some calming breaths and think about something happy to pass the time. You may also try to meditate if that will help relax you.

The typical schedule will likely involve one longer appointment a week and four short ones. The long appointments include a visit with your radiation oncologist. He or she will examine your skin and check on your overall health. The exams are relatively brief, but you do need to allow some extra time for them. You may also get X-rays taken about once a week to double-check that the radiation is getting to the right spots.

The other days of the week, you can probably expect to spend about fifteen minutes or less in radiation, depending on your individual prescription. Of course, the entire process of parking, changing, and waiting will take a bit longer.

Most people can expect a treatment schedule of five to seven weeks. You may also hear about a radiation boost at the end of your treatment. That refers to several additional treatments to the area where the tumor was removed.

KELLEY: I did okay on the first day of radiation. It wasn't so bad and didn't hurt. But as I've said before, I was pretty emotionally fragile by the time I got to radiation. I had endured seven months of hell including surgery and chemo, and I was exhausted. On my second day of radiation, I started to cry as I left the machine. I just felt like a cow being herded through this horrible radiation mill. I hated rushing out of my house before the kids woke up, then rushing to radiation so I could then rush to work. At night I would go to bed and do it all over again the next day. My *Groundhog Day* was a horror movie.

I was petrified someone was going to call a social worker to deal with this basket case on the radiation floor. Instead, a loving radiation therapist who had been helping women like me for thirty years knew just what to do. Joan looked me in the eye and said, "We're here for you. Anything you need, we're here to help." It was perfect. I felt reassured I was in good hands with people who help women every day. I said thank you and went home with a new determination to get through this with strength and grace. What did the little engine say? I think I can, I think I can.

FAMILIAR FACES

You may find a lot of encouragement from the other women who will become part of your radiation experience. You will come to know their stories and their friends and families. It's an interesting and unusual experience to bond with so many women whom you will see only for a few minutes each day. You will celebrate as each of them "graduates" from radiation and heads off to what you hope will be a long, healthy life.

Elisha was incredibly touched by the amazing women she met in the radiation waiting room. Everyone was so strong and provided encouragement to one another. On Elisha's last day of radiation the ladies presented her with a cake and a long-stemmed, hot-pink silk flower. Elisha keeps that flower on her office desk where she can see it every day to remember those women who were strangers but became loving friends.

Sanity Saver

Try to avoid doing too much cancer-comparison talk in the radiation waiting area. It's very stressful to hear what treatment program one person has that you may not be getting. Everyone's cancers are different, and there may be a good reason for different protocols. Try to keep conversation light if possible.

BE A PATIENT PATIENT

Radiation can become very disruptive to your schedule, especially if you can't get a time slot you like. Consider getting radiation on your lunch break or at the end of the day. Maybe there's a time when your kids are at school that might work. Do the best you can to take some of the stress out of fitting in this very important treatment.

Even then, prepare yourself for the inevitable delay days. If you are lucky, you won't encounter any problems. But machines break down, and radiation centers get backed up. Find out if there's a way you can check on whether things are on schedule before you leave your home. Many centers will call you if there's a big problem. Make sure your nurses and radiation therapists have your cell phone number so they can easily reach you.

ELISHA: I knew I needed to get myself in the earliest time slot possible. I figured if I could get in for treatment at 7 or 7:30 a.m., I could get out in time to have a full uninterrupted, cancer-free day. Also, the earlier in the day you get in for treatment, the less likely you'll be delayed if the radiation machines get backed up as the day goes on.

I was so accustomed to a crazy, busy schedule that it was extremely hard for me to be tied to the hospital every morning. I was used to traveling all over the country, being in New York City a couple days a week and basically never sitting still. If patience is not your strong suit, then radiation will definitely be a challenge for you. Waiting around is a big part of these weeks. As much as I refused to allow breast cancer to get the better of my time or energy, I had to concede to the fact that I had to respect the importance of my treatment. Radiation was designed to save my life.

Every week I would go for radiation at 7 a.m. and still make the 9:20 train to New York City, work all day, and catch the 5 or 6 o'clock train home just to do it all over again the next morning. It was not my ideal schedule, but at least I had some control over my life. I remember halfway through my radiation treatment I got the opportunity to present the clothing line to Neiman Marcus in Dallas. It would mean missing a day of treatment, but there was no way I was going to let this opportunity pass me by. I discussed my situation with my doctor and he allowed me to make up the missed day at the end of treatment.

SIDE EFFECTS

You probably won't want to or be able to keep up that type of schedule. Your fatigue might be more problematic depending on your age, your level of fitness, and your general health. The burns may be uncomfortable. If you are used to leading a high-energy lifestyle, radiation fatigue can be frustrating. Dr. Wong says there's no way to predict who will suffer from fatigue. Most patients are somewhat tired but able to function, but others report debilitating pain. Every patient is different, and you have to be patient with yourself.

Radiation does come with some other side effects. Skin burns are the most common. Elisha had no direct side effects related to radiation, with the exception of fatigue as the weeks went by. She is very fair skinned, so she took great precautions to prevent any burning or irritation on her skin. Although doctors say there are no magic creams to avoid burns, Elisha decided to try PCA Skin products. She would layer their ReBalance Cream and Silkcoat Balm over her skin nightly.

Kelley used Aquaphor nightly but still got a pretty nasty burn. It was itchy and uncomfortable. And the greasy lotion stained a few of her shirts! The burn went away a few months after she finished treatment, and the skin in that area is pretty much back to normal. Kelley also struggled with fatigue but never quite knew if it was the radiation, the punishing schedule, or residual fatigue from chemo.

There are a few important things to remember during radiation. First, avoid all sun exposure. Make sure you wear a lot of sunscreen. Keep radiation areas covered from the sun when possible. Avoid wearing deodorant before treatment. It can interfere with radiation or worsen the skin's reaction. Eat healthy foods and drink a lot of water. Your radiation oncologist may recommend a multivitamin. And keep exercising to combat fatigue, a common side effect from this treatment.

For us, the most difficult part was just being at the hospital every day. It's a pain to get there and annoying to wait. Bring a book to read or work to do while you wait around. Anything that takes your mind off why you are there helps save your sanity. Also, wear comfortable clothes. That doesn't mean lose your style—just be comfortable. Try wearing soft, lightweight undergarments that won't scratch your irritated skin. Maybe a silk or cotton camisole will be more comfortable than a bra with underwire.

Radiation ultimately was a major inconvenience at the end of the year from hell. We tried to remind ourselves that we were in a fight for our lives. Focusing on the big picture may help you get past the impatience you may feel by the daily rigors of this treatment. Take care of your skin, get plenty of sleep, and try to stay positive. See if you can convince a friend or two to come with you to break up the monotony. Six weeks is a long time, but you can get through it.

Don't Lose Your Sanity!

- Get a big calendar and cross off the days for encouragement.
- Think of some great reward—big or small—for your last day.
- Take care of yourself. If fatigue is a problem, find time for a nap. And make sure you exercise and eat right.
- Consider complementary therapies such as yoga, massage, or Reiki to help with side effects.

Don't Lose Your Style!

- Keep the radiation area moisturized!
- Wear sunscreen and avoid exposure to radiation area.
- Invest in some pretty silk or cotton camisoles that feel soft against your skin.
- Get your beauty rest—it's okay to give in to your fatigue.

Lose the Cancer, Not Your Style

most of us are used to feeling like we have a strong sense of self and some control over our lives. Cancer tries to strip you of these qualities, but you cannot give in to feeling powerless. Take charge! You may reach a point in treatment when you pass a mirror and have no idea who the person is looking back at you. Trust us, we both work in the public eye where appearance matters. And we both needed and wanted to keep working and living life as we knew it.

Call it survival of the chicest! No matter how awful you feel inside, knowing you look fabulous on the outside is sure to make you feel better. There are proven psychological benefits to looking your best while feeling your worst. Cancer treatment wreaks havoc on your body and your looks, but if you make an effort to keep up your appearance and style, you will feel better and look less like a cancer patient. As crazy as it may sound, fashion and beauty can inspire you to never give up.

If you look healthy, people will treat you like your old self instead of like a cancer patient. It's a cycle that leads to the beginning of better days ahead.

Kelley continued to work on air at WCVB-TV in Boston throughout treatment. She tried to keep up her appearance at all times, but once she arrived at the station on a Sunday with no makeup on. It was about eight months into treatment.

KELLEY: Without my wig and makeup I didn't recognize myself in the mirror anymore. To make matters worse, I had several incidents where people I know didn't recognize me. It made me feel even more like a freak show. On that Sunday when I didn't wear makeup, a coworker actually introduced himself to me. He said, "Sorry, I didn't know it was you." I replied, "Of course not. I'm wearing a wig, and I have no eyebrows and no eyelashes." Why would anyone recognize me when I could barely recognize myself?

Sanity Saver

Run, don't walk to the nearest Look Good . . . Feel Better program (http://www.lookgoodfeelbetter.org, or 800-395-LOOK). These workshops are available across the country and offer specific advice on how to best use makeup and head coverings to improve your appearance during treatment. It's a free program run by professionals who have extensive experience dealing with cancer patients.

BROWS

Elisha's eyebrows thinned but did not completely fall out. Kelley's dark, thick brows were decimated. It really changed her look and aged her tremendously.

Eyebrows are important because they shape and define your face. When shaped properly, they can open up your eyes. If you lose them, not only is it a shock to you visually, it is also one more reminder that you really are a cancer patient.

Estée Lauder global makeup stylist Rick DiCecca has worked with such renowned beauties as Cindy Crawford, Iman, and Heidi Klum. But he's most proud of what he's done for some of his special clients: helping women battling cancer feel like supermodels in their own right. We asked him to explain the secret to creating a natural-looking eyebrow.

He says secret to creating a perfect brow is one line and two dots. Place a long thin object such as a brow pencil or makeup brush alongside of your nose and make a small vertical mark or line in front of the pencil or brush in line with the brow. Now, looking straight ahead, roll the pencil or brush in front of the eye until it lines up with the outer edge of the pupil; make a dot on the skin along the brow bone. Finally, using the bottom edge of the nose and the outer corner of the eye as guides, place the last dot in line with the first.

Using an eye pencil, start at the bottom of the small vertical mark and draw a line up to the first dot. Then draw a second line from the top of the mark to the first dot and a third line from the first dot to the last, connecting all. Go back and fill in the area at the beginning of the brow with featherlike strokes.

If you need more help, try going to a salon for a consultation. A professional can show you simple steps you can take to create an eyebrow. You can also pick up eyebrow kits at your local beauty supply store or order them online. Fill-in stencil kits might work for you. You just put the stencil over your brow and fill in with a pencil. You can also check out stick-on prosthetic eyebrows to see if that may be a better option for your face.

Kelley's eyebrows did come back, but they weren't exactly like they were precancer. She now has thin spots on her once thick brows. That eyebrow pencil is now a permanent part of her makeup kit.

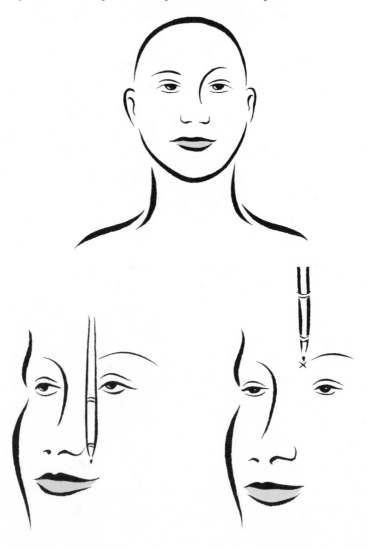

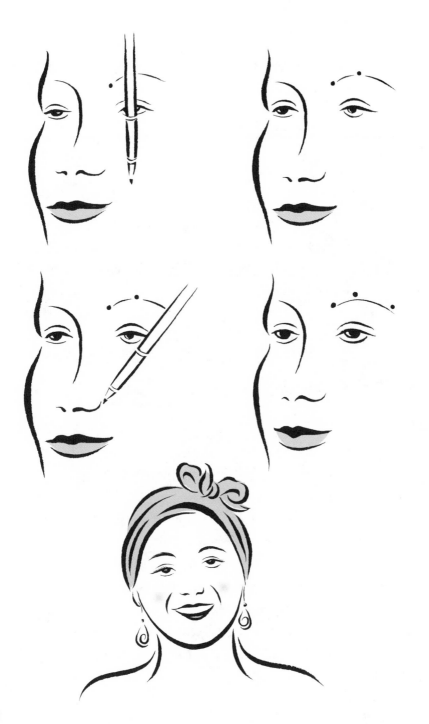

LASHES

There is something about losing your eyelashes that really makes you look like a cancer patient. Lashes give a lot of definition to our eyes.

ELISHA: As hard as it was to lose my hair, I think it was worse when my eyelashes started to fall out. That happened around my fourth or fifth Taxol treatment, which was approximately the halfway point. I continued to put mascara on them until every last one was gone. I remember having one long lash in the middle of my right eye and I put mascara on it. I tried to do false lashes, but I was no good at it. I had this vision of them falling off into my food during a dinner party, or one hanging off the corner of my eye when I was talking to someone. Again, they just didn't look real to me, so I opted for nothing. I did discover a way to create the illusion of lashes with an eye pencil. I penciled in my top lid between my lid and my lash bed, which gave the illusion of lashes. It works!

Rick DiCecca agrees. He says, "The trick to getting great-looking eyes is to use a dark eyeliner in black, brown, or gray and apply it very close to the edge of the upper lid, smudging it to create soft definition in the area where lashes were. You may apply a coordinating eye shadow over the eyeliner to set and to increase wear time."

When Kelley's lashes started to go she decided to try professional lash extensions. They were beautiful and made her eyes pop from an increasingly sallow face. Unfortunately, when she went back a month or so later, the salon had to turn Kelley away. You actually have to have some eyelashes in order to attach the extensions. Kelley had none. She was devastated.

KELLEY: During radiation, I was asked to fill in anchoring the early morning newscast. I had no hair, no eyelashes, and no eyebrows. It was definitely easier to hide my appearance issues in my two-minute reporting segments. But for a two-hour show there was no place to hide.

I arrived at 3 a.m. to do everything I needed to do to look presentable. (FYI: We do our own makeup at the station!) The wig needed to be on just right. But then I had to do the brows and lashes. Brows I could manage okay, but lashes? OMG. I was barely awake and struggling with glue and sticky fingers. Not easy at all. It's a wonder I made it on air. But I was determined the show would go on despite treatment, and it did. I used a lot of teeth whitening strips that week. Something had to sparkle! Most important, I still had my years of journalism experience, my education, and my personality. Cancer did not take my strong foundation away. I had to reach deep inside me to find the strength and confidence to get through that uncomfortable and challenging situation.

If you decide to go with false eyelashes, you can either go to a professional or do it yourself. Going to a salon or specialty shop will cost you more, but it is something to consider if you've never put on false lashes before. You could really hurt your eyes with the adhesive if you don't know what you are doing. Plus, a professional will help you achieve the most natural look. The other option is to get a do-it-yourself kit at your local drugstore or beauty store.

Immediately after her chemo treatments were finished, Elisha's hair and lashes began to grow back. You may find your lashes and hair will grow back thicker than ever. But Elisha found that every once in a while, up to a year after her treatment, her lashes would start to fall out again.

Dr. Partridge says that's because lashes fall out on a regular basis and when they all fall out with chemo, apparently the clock gets reset. When they grow back, many of them are cycling together rather than at different times. Some women even lose all of their lashes for a second time before things go back to normal.

NAILS

You may notice some strange changes to your nails. They may become discolored or brittle or both! The good news is that your chemo drugs are working right down to your toenails. Fortunately, these changes are usually temporary. The best advice we can give you is to take good care of your nails in the meantime.

Keep nails short so they won't break off. Keep your hands and nails well moisturized. A little vitamin E or olive oil rubbed on your nails at night really helps.

A manicure and pedicure will help hide ugly discoloration. Do not try to buff or file off streaks or spots; this can damage your nails. When you polish your nails, just push back cuticles instead of cutting them. You don't want to put yourself at risk for an infection.

You may also want to avoid artificial nails right now. The chemical adhesives can cause even more damage to your fragile nails.

ELISHA: I have always taken good care of my nails—I get a weekly manicure and a monthly pedicure. My fingernails were fine throughout treatment, but my toenails on my right foot all turned brown and fell off. I was completely freaked out and horrified. This was definitely not a good look in my Jimmy Choo stiletto sandals. But just like every other unattractive, uncomfortable change that comes on this journey, I survived the toenail episode. And, like everything else, they actually grew back fine.

SKIN CARE

You may find one day you wake up and the color of your skin has changed. Some people will even look gray. You will want to take good care of your skin, including using gentle cleansers, because your skin may be more sensitive. Rick DiCecca says, "My best advice for women to regain their healthy glow is to find and use a great moisturizer. You need one that not only hydrates but also revitalizes the skin and creates luminosity."

Keeping skin hydrated has to come from within as well. Make sure you drink a lot of water every day. You will feel and look better if you do.

You also might want to experiment with tinted moisturizers or bronzers to see if they can perk up your dull complexion.

THE CLOTHES ON YOUR BACK

Style is not about the clothes on your back; it is an extension of your confidence, your spirit, and your positive attitude—all the same attributes that will help you survive breast cancer with sanity and style.

During this extremely challenging time in your life, your focus should certainly be on getting healthy, but there is no reason to sacrifice your style. You don't have to sit in the infusion room in a depressing old tracksuit. There are some wonderful clothing lines out there that will keep you looking chic and confident.

In our lives both professionally and socially, we are always out in public. Neither one of us had any intention of going into hibernation just because we were fighting breast cancer. But you might want to plan on spending a little more time and effort to get ready every morning. Put on your lipstick, straighten your wig or your scarf, and get on with your day.

If you are having trouble finding clothes that look right on your surgically altered body, check out Chikara (http://www.chikaradesign.com), a clothing collection that effortlessly balances the body following breast cancer treatments and surgeries. They achieve a balanced look through asymmetrical and three-dimensional design. Chikara allows women to embrace their sense of style by choosing from pieces that are inspired by their body types.

You can also go shopping in your own closet. Be creative! Take some comfortable basics, such as a classic white shirt, black pencil skirt, or black cigarette pants, and update it with accessories. We both tend to opt for color because it's so uplifting, but classic black and white is always crisp and easy to pull together.

ELISHA: I have been the stylist for many fashion shows, including many style shows on QVC, and I promise you, you will always get compliments wearing black and white. I also found that dressing in layers was very helpful. Chemo pushed me into early menopause, and suddenly I was dealing with constant hot flashes. One minute I was roasting, the next minute I was freezing. Dressing in layers provided the option of taking clothes on and off to be comfortable.

A LITTLE LIFT

In the midst of all this, you may want to take time to go bra shopping. You may be wearing a prosthesis or have expanders or a new reconstruction in place. Either way your old bras probably don't fit like they used to. A good bra will help make sure your clothes hang right. Head to a lingerie store and get a proper fitting so you can be comfortable. There are now a lot of options when it comes to bra shopping, and many stores specialize in getting the perfect fit. We love Intimacy (http://www.myintimacy.com) and Nordstrom's lingerie department (http://www.nordstroms.com). This is one "lift" that might make you feel instantly better.

ELISHA: I will never forget being in New York City visiting one of my oldest friends. One morning I had a little time to kill, so I stopped into my favorite Italian café on the Upper East Side for a latte. I sat down at a table with my newspaper, minding my own business. Within minutes the guy next to me was trying to chat with me and, for lack of a better word, hitting on me. I couldn't help feeling that this was a wonderful compliment because in my own mind I was thinking, "Mister, if you only knew you are hitting on a bald chick with one boob, you'd run a mile!"

To be honest, we can't promise you that you will ever get comfortable with how you look during this time. But we *can* promise you that a huge part of getting through this moment is knowing that these challenges are only temporary. You are in control of how you look. You can work to hide the effects of cancer or let the world know you are fighting for your life. You do it your way without fear of what anyone else thinks. Think of FEAR as "False Events Appearing Real." Look at this stage of your recovery for what it is, and don't forget that your hair and your eyelashes and your eyebrows will come back. You will look like you again soon.

Don't Lose Your Sanity!

- Be kind to yourself. Beating the cancer is the most important thing.
- Get professional help with your appearance if you need it. There are many wonderful hair, makeup, and clothing stylists who have experience with breast cancer patients. And Look Good . . . Feel Better is free!

Don't Lose Your Style!

- Experiment with makeup, clothes, and hair accessories.
- Play around with tinted moisturizers and bronzers. They may help perk up a dull complexion.
- Treat yourself to a gentle facial to relax you and improve your skin tone.
- Find your most comfortable look and wear it with confidence.
- Make your own cancer fashion statements.

Help!

It's an incredibly humbling experience to go from leading an independent life to being dependent on others. You may come to treasure your family and friends more than you ever thought possible. People want to help you get through this, and you need to let them!

Depending on your treatment regime, you or your family may need friends and loved ones to support you physically and emotionally. Since we were little girls, we have both been fiercely independent. Our parents raised us to take care of ourselves and support ourselves. We never expected to find ourselves in such a vulnerable and scary position. There were many days when we felt weak and scared. But it was the support of friends and loved ones that often made us feel safe and secure again.

There are a lot of hard lessons learned on this journey. You may find that some well-intentioned people will burden you with their own emotional needs and concerns about your illness. You will need to figure out how to protect yourself from this. Sometimes the people you think are going to be there for you let you down, and people who were merely acquaintances become trusted, lifelong friends.

MANAGE THE INFORMATION

Early on you may want to appoint someone you trust to be your spokesperson, so to speak. It can be a burden to tell your cancer stories and give updates over and over again, even to caring family and friends. A spokesperson can be in charge of spreading the information you want to get out to the masses.

One suggestion is to have a friend set up an account on a Web site such as http://www.carepages.com or http://www.caringbridge.org. It's a great way to manage the flow of information. You can either update the page yourself or ask your spokesperson to do it for you. You can post updates at key points, such as when you are out of surgery and want to let everyone know you are okay.

There's also a place for people to post notes of encouragement. It's kind of nice to have these postings in a separate place where you can read them when you are in the mood. Having constant e-mails filling your mailbox can be overwhelming. Postings on a separate Web site can provide a source of support and connection with the outside world without the burden of feeling like a response is required. These Web sites are an easy way to keep people near and far updated on how you are doing. You may also find it comforting to write about your experiences and share them with others. It may be good way for you to process all you are going through.

MANAGE THE HELP

Of course, one of the things people might ask you is "How can I help?" Another great Web site to look into is http://www.lotsahelpinghands.com. This site allows you to list what might be helpful, and then your family and friends can sign up for tasks. It's an easy way to ensure you don't get three lasagnas on one night. You can post anything, from a ride to the cancer center to helping with the children's carpools to meals. It's a great way to ask others for help without ever having to directly ask.

If you have children in your home, chances are you are going to need help during cancer treatment. It may be just too hard to handle all your usual responsibilities while getting treated for cancer with all the potential side effects. To accept that help, you will certainly have to get used to giving up some control over your life. And that's not easy.

Sanity Saver

Even if you coordinate everything online, consider getting a big calendar and placing it in a prominent spot in your home. It's a good way for all involved to make sure meals, rides, and other essentials are kept straight. It also ensures that older kids and husbands know what to expect.

SPEAK UP

Try to get comfortable being direct with people about what you find helpful or annoying. If that is too hard for you then give the job to someone who can handle it. We all have a bossy friend or relative. If someone is offering to take your children and you would rather have them with you, speak up! If someone starts to clean your house and you don't want them to, tell them maybe later.

People often ask us how to best help a woman going through treatment. Here are some ideas:

- Hang out with her and be good, easy company. Be sensitive to her mood. Maybe she needs to talk about cancer, but maybe she needs to talk about anything else.
- Don't overreact, cry, or act like she's dying.
- Do something nice for her kids to make them feel special.
- Volunteer to drive kids to school or activities. Make kids' lunches if appropriate. (This is a great way for a school community to help a family in need.)
- Have your husband take her husband out for a beer or to a sporting event.
- Offer to go away with her for a night or longer.
- Offer to clean or do laundry.
- Offer to go to a medical appointment or treatment.
- Volunteer to drive to radiation one day and wait in the car so she doesn't have to park for the twentieth time!
- Fill her iPod with great music to lift her spirits.
- Arrange a girl's outing—dinner, a spa day, or shopping.
- Take-out gift certificates or grocery store cards can be very helpful.
- In some circumstances, a cash gift may be appropriate to help a family cope with the unending expenses of a major illness.

And we hate to say it, but here are some don'ts:
- Don't say, "Let me know if there's anything I can do." (That puts it back on the patient to ask for something. A specific offer is always better and seems more sincere.)
- Never drop in unannounced at a cancer patient's house. You just never know what's going on at that moment.
- Never assume the patient can't do something or won't be interested. We want to be included and treated like we're still alive!

- Don't take over a household or child-care duty without clearing it with the patient. It may just make her feel more powerless rather than empowered by loving help and kindness.

Saying Thanks

It can be overwhelming to think about thanking people for all the kind things they will do for you during treatment. Don't worry if it takes you a while to send thank-you notes. People understand you have a lot going on, and they will give you a pass. But if you would like to, here are some ideas for acknowledging the kindness around you.

- Ask your closest friends or family to help you address envelopes.
- Consider making a standard letter on your computer with a heartfelt note thanking people for their thoughtfulness. That way you can just print it out as needed.
- You can always just make a master list of acts of kindness and send thank-you notes at the end of the year.
- E-mail is fine if you don't feel up to writing thank-you notes. People understand.
- Consider making your holiday card double as a thank-you to all those who have helped you and your family.

A Humbling Experience

We have both met a lot of amazing people throughout our cancer journeys. Kelley met Mindy Wanatick, an extraordinary woman who put up an incredibly tough fight against brain cancer. Her father, George Millington, wrote an e-mail to family and friends that really captures how touching it can be to have family, friends, and strangers reach out in your time of need.

Those who have not had the chance to experience the immutable kind-ness, generosity, and selflessness of dear, loyal friends have missed out on one of life's greatest gifts.

You have taught us that to be human and suffering is to be part of a vibrant, cohesive community that truly cares. Our pain has become your shared pain; our burden has been eased by your bearing it with us. Knowing this serves to diffuse an intolerable situation, and make it one that is manageable, albeit difficult. Your extraordinary loving embrace of Mindy as she fights to stay alive each day for her husband and children simply overwhelms us with its powerful message of love and hope. We will never, ever forget what you have done for us.

Many of us could probably write the same words to our incredible sup-porters. That feeling of love and support is truly a gift from this horrible disease.

Giving Back

One way to cope with the overwhelming emotions you may be feeling is to think about ways you might want to give back when you're ready. For some women, participating in a big weekend walk or a smaller breast cancer walk can be a great way to connect with other survivors and help worthy causes.

You can volunteer at the cancer center where you were treated if you feel you can handle that. You could agree to mentor a newly diagnosed patient.

Within your community there may be organizations big and small that provide outreach to women in treatment. In Boston, the Ellie Fund pro-vides meals, transportation, and house cleaning to breast cancer patients. Kelley has worked with that charity and many others to ease the impact on other women and help find a cure. She has also used her role as a newscaster to do stories and raise awareness about early detection. She also speaks publicly about her painful experience to help others.

Elisha has used her talents to help the Breast Cancer Research Foundation (BCRF) (http://www.bcrfcure.org), a charity that funds exciting research at institutions across the country. Elisha and designer Sara Campbell (http://www.saracampbell.com) have created signature shirts, bags, and scarves with a portion of the proceeds going to BCRF. They have also hosted fashion shows featuring survivors, all to benefit this charity.

ELISHA: Halfway through my chemo treatment, I was in Palm Beach on a short vacation. I was invited to a fabulous, swanky party at a friend's home. I wore a wonderful party dress with a coordinating Hermes scarf on my bald head, but there was no hiding that I was a cancer patient. That night I was introduced to Sandy Krakoff, a woman who would change my life. We connected immediately and spent hours chatting about cancer treatments, doctors, and research.

My new friend turned out to be an amazing source of inspiration for me. She supported me throughout my breast cancer treatment, then within months after my treatment was complete, her husband died suddenly and she was diagnosed with breast cancer herself. The irony of this tragedy is that this is a woman who has spent her life giving money and raising money for cancer research. Now she unexpectedly had to join our club. I was so inspired by her that I started raising hundreds of thousands of dollars to help fund research.

It was the first time since I had been diagnosed that I was on the other side. Suddenly I was in the position to support and help someone I had come to admire and love. I had the opportunity to give back the support that had been given to me by so many friends and loved ones. There is something empowering about being able to support someone else with your hard-earned knowledge. The unfortunate part is that since then I have had the opportunity to help more friends than I wish to count, which means more women than ever are being struck by cancer.

Myra Biblowit, the president of BCRF, always says she will be happy the day her charity is out of business. That will mean breast cancer is cured and there is no more need for research. As impossible as that may seem, we believe that day is getting closer and closer. We may see that day in our lifetime. We all have to work together for a cure so that Kelley's girls, Madeline and Cecilia, and all young girls never have to endure what we went through.

There is no denying that surviving breast cancer changes your life forever. You may want to give back to all the people and organizations that helped save your life. You simply can't give back to everyone, but you can do your part. It doesn't have to be a monetary contribution. Maybe you can volunteer your time, lead a support group, or sign up for a walk or run.

We have tried to use our unique talents and interests to help conquer cancer. It's so empowering to find an outlet for the frustration you feel at having to join a club you never wanted to be a member of.

Don't Lose Your Sanity!

- Appoint someone to coordinate both updates and offers of help.
- Don't forget that it's still your life and your house. Speak up if you are unhappy or feel like you are losing control.

- Don't stress over thank-you notes. When you are up to it, write a heartfelt e-mail or something simple on your computer. People understand you have other things on your plate.

Don't Lose Your Style!

- Don't turn your back on what you have been through. Use your experience to help someone else when and if you are ready.
- Find your niche within an organization and give back what you can.
- Embrace the new friends you've met along the way. Remember they are the gifts from this difficult experience.
- Remember your true beauty comes from within and is only enhanced by the lessons learned along this journey.

TEN

Kids, Couples, Careers, and Other Challenges

ancer, as you have probably realized, does not just affect the patient; it affects everyone around her. This one diagnosis can impact your family, friends, coworkers, and community. Unless you have children, it's not necessarily your problem to help others cope. But you may want to think about how best to deal with all the chaos that may come with your diagnosis.

We all have our priorities in life. Whether it's your children, your career, your church, or community service, these are the things that drive you. That is, until you are diagnosed with breast cancer. Suddenly those priorities have to shift a little. Now your number one priority has to be gearing up for the biggest fight of your life! And you thought you juggled a lot before cancer? Ha! Life is about to get a lot more complicated. But we know you have it in you to keep it all together (at least most days). You can do this!

Kids

For parents of dependent children a cancer diagnosis takes on a whole new dimension. We may worry about how our cancer will affect our parents, partners, and friends, but children must have our special consideration.

In chapter 1, we discussed how best to share the news of your diagnosis with your children. The key is to be honest and direct. You may be surprised how little they want to talk about it when you first introduce the topic. If you sense they have had enough information for one sitting, allow the conversation to come to its natural conclusion. You can then wait for questions as they come.

One way to spark a conversation with children is to ask them questions about how they perceive your disease and treatment. That way you can make sure they are handling everything okay.

Here are some basic parenting tips:

- Let your children know what's going on and what will happen next. If appropriate, offer some hope that there will be better times ahead.
- Find a quiet time to talk with your children. Listen to their fears and let them ask questions. Validate their feelings and let them know it's okay to feel sad, angry, or confused.
- Assure your kids that they will be cared for and loved.
- Remind children that cancer is not contagious, and that nothing they did caused your disease.
- Correct any misconceptions your children may have. Asking questions is a good way to figure out what they are thinking.
- Try not to make promises you may not be able to keep. Instead say, "I think I can" or "I'll try to."
- Keep your family's routines intact when possible and try to minimize disruptions.
- Keep schools and your pediatrician up to date about what's going on.

Dr. Paula Rauch founded the Parenting at a Challenging Time, or PACT, program at Massachusetts General Hospital and is the author of *Raising an Emotionally Healthy Child When a Parent Is Sick*. Kelley's coworker gave her this book after her diagnosis. Kelley eventually had a chance to speak with Dr. Rauch, who really helped her with her parenting concerns. We asked Dr. Rauch to answer some of the key questions many parents have.

Q: **Any advice for people who simply cannot find the words to tell their children about a breast cancer diagnosis?**

A: Even for children as young as three years old, there are no better words to use than, "I have breast cancer." Using terms such "lump," "bump," or even "a growth" are more likely to confuse your child. Young children may have lumps and bumps themselves and worry that they will need the same intense treatment you may receive and perhaps lose their hair, too. Older children may feel lied to when they later learn that your medical condition is breast cancer, not whatever general term you may have used to gloss over the actual diagnosis.

When you use the real term "breast cancer," you allow your child to talk about your cancer and to learn about it. Indirect communication and euphemisms leave children to get their information by overhearing adult conversations or hearing the news from other family or friends. This is the worst way to hear significant information. It may convey to your child that the topic of cancer is too scary to be discussed directly, or it may leave your child feeling excluded from serious conversations, because she is not as important as the people who are receiving the parent's direct communication. Remember, exclusion from a caring conversation should never be imagined as protective. It leaves children to wonder and worry alone.

Q: **How do you start the conversation?**

A: Many parents find it hard to start the conversation, because they feel as if sharing this unwelcome news is hurtful to the child. Research shows that though children acknowledge that learning about a parent's cancer is upsetting, they always want to know and appreciate being included in this important family experience.

   During the days or weeks leading up to your cancer diagnosis, there likely have been some observable changes at home affecting your child. You can begin the conversation by asking your child what he or she has noticed that is different or by describing these recent events yourself. Examples of conversation starters might be, "You know I've been going to the doctor for appointments (or Grandma is coming for a special visit, or Daddy and I have been having lots of grown-up talks)," or "Have you noticed that I have been on the phone more than usual?" Younger children will usually find this narrative helpful. Older children may become upset on hearing the news, so you may want to pick a quiet time and a private place to begin the conversation. It will be important to ask them what they are most worried about so that you can address their specific concerns.

Q: **What if your child asks if you are going to die?**

A: Some parents are so afraid of being asked about the possibility of dying that it is hard to discuss the breast cancer diagnosis at all. In most cases, breast cancer is discovered at a time when there are good treatment options for you. If this is the case, letting your child know that while it is true that women can die from breast cancer, your doctors are not worried about you dying now, but are focused on what is the best treatment for your kind of breast cancer. It is helpful to let children know that there are many different types of breast cancer and there are different stages, so that other people's breast cancer experiences cannot predict your own. To learn about your medical situation, your child needs to ask you specific questions and hear answers directly from you and perhaps your spouse. Let your child know that as you receive news, you will share it.

Q: What are the most important things you can do for your child during treatment?

A: Parents will want to focus on three areas that support a child's best ways to cope at times of stress. One is to keep routines and schedules as consistent as possible. This may mean keeping younger children on their preexisting eating and sleeping schedules. Fewer consistent caregivers are easier for young children to feel safe with and easier for parents to partner with to keep things as normal as possible. Older children will have school and after-school activities that can help them reestablish a sense of normalcy. A smaller number of favorite activities attended regularly are better than more activities and spotty attendance. Teachers should be informed about the parent's medical situation and encouraged to notify parents of any concerns. Most children will want school to be an oasis away from medical concerns and will not want their mother's breast cancer discussed with classmates, but it is always best to ask your child what he or she would want. Children should know which adult they can go to at school if they have a problem or worry related to their mother's illness or treatment.

The second is to protect family time and keep the focus on the children during those key times. This often means asking friends not to call or visit during dinnertime and being available to your child after school and before bedtime. If parents can continue to provide help with homework, show interest in a child's daily experiences, and plan some fun family times, children can continue to feel good about their family. Feeling lucky to be a part of a loving family is always important.

The third important area is communication between children and parents and parents and children. Good communication begins with good listening. Parents should learn to listen and listen to learn. When children sense that a parent is really interested in what they think and feel, they are much more likely to share their thoughts and feelings. Welcome your child's ideas and questions with warmth and curiosity. Say things such as, "That's a really interesting idea," or "What a good question. It really makes me think."

Encourage children to elaborate their thoughts and questions with comments such as, "What got you wondering about that?" or "Help me understand which part you are most upset about." It is helpful to remember that children's questions need not be answered immediately. It can be very respectful to tell a child that to answer the question well means talking with another adult, such as another parent, doctor, or clergy person, or looking the information up in a quality resource. Most parents know the times and places that their children are mostly likely to have thoughtful conversations. Amid the many hectic demands of cancer treatment, it is helpful to be mindful of those reflective times and to make it a priority to protect those special times with your child when possible.

Some children talk easily, and others seem to keep most of their thoughts and feelings to themselves. Check in with every child and ask if there are any lingering worries, frustrations, or confusion about your treatment. Make sure your child knows what the side effects of your treatment are and that they are not evidence of advancing disease. Finally, remind your child that you are checking in because you do not want her to worry alone. When children feel well loved and connected with their parents during challenging times, they learn important life skills that will serve them well as they face new challenges in the future.

KELLEY'S CHILDREN

Kelley's girls were just two and a half and six months old when cancer invaded their happy lives. Kelley tried to be as up-front with Madeline as possible. Just before her mastectomy, Kelley sat down with Maddie and told her that Mommy had breast cancer and would need an operation. Maddie had very little to say and quickly asked what was for dinner. But throughout treatment Maddie did have questions, and Kelley and Brendan did their best to provide simple, straightforward answers.

KELLEY: It was actually very difficult because I struggled as Maddie turned three to know how much I should include her in my experience and how much I should protect her. She was very interested in my hair loss. I think it really threw her off to see me without hair. She knew that wasn't normal. I had to keep reassuring her that it wouldn't happen to her. I had to make sure she knew regular medicine did not make people's hair fall out.

Maddie did visit me in the hospital postsurgery, and that went very well. We cuddled and watched a movie and she didn't seem too upset to see me in that setting. I never let her come to chemo, but I did let her join me for some radiation sessions. Maddie would come into the hospital with me and sit in the waiting area while I got radiation. The other women would dote on her, and she loved the attention. It gave us an extra hour to spend together.

This part of treatment proved very difficult on my husband and little girls. It messed up our entire routine. Halfway through treatment Brendan looked at me and said, "This really isn't working for me." I wanted to club him over the head, but I knew what he meant. It wasn't really working for any of us. He liked to head to work early every day. I liked taking the kids to school. Everything was upside down.

So Maddie came to radiation maybe a half dozen times. I'm not sure if it was the right call. Perhaps I should have protected her from the sickness more. There's no rule book. You just do the best you can given your family's circumstances. She missed me and wanted to be with me. I missed her. By the end of radiation, though, I was growing concerned she was focusing too much on taking care of me. I had to work to rebalance the relationship so I could be her caregiver again, not the other way around.

The hardest moment I ever had with Maddie happened during the final day of radiation. Brendan, Maddie, and Cecie all came and we brought coffee and doughnuts for the other patients and staff. I was so overwhelmed by the end of treatment that I started to cry. They were really tears of joy because I was so happy to be done. Maddie was very confused and talked for weeks about when Mommy cried. Nothing I said could convince her I was happy to be done with the hospital. All she remembered was seeing Mom cry. You may have these moments where you, too, will struggle with how much to protect or include your children in your cancer experience.

The most important thing is to continuously check in to see how they are processing what they observe. Cancer treatment brings so many ups and downs; it's virtually impossible to protect your kids from everything. And protecting them may not always be the best idea anyway.

There are resources in your community to help you make the best decisions about your kids. Your hospital social worker deals with these situations all the time. He or she should be able to offer solid advice. The American Cancer Society sponsors many different programs, some specifically for children of patients. If you live near a Wellness Community location (http://www.thewellnesscommunity.org), check out their offerings. And don't forget the resources at your children's schools. Sadly, you are not the first parent to cope with a cancer diagnosis. Teachers should be notified of your family's situation and contacted should problems arise.

One of the best things you can do for a child is to keep his or her routine as normal as possible. This is not always easy, especially if you were the primary person who coordinated your children's lives. It's not going to be normal if Mom doesn't drive to school like she always does. Just make sure you have a solid plan in place and communicate it to your children. They will want to know what to expect. They will want to be reassured that they will be taken care of at all times. Children, though wonderfully caring, tend to be rather self-centered and to worry about how all this will affect them.

One thing Kelley wished she had been stronger about was keeping a routine during the height of her crisis, so to speak. Right after surgery and during those early chemo days, people would stop by at various times. The house was always bustling with people and ringing doorbells and phones. It did not feel like precancer life.

Kelley admits that she needed the distraction and the interaction to keep her mind off the disease and treatment. But for the kids and Brendan, all that noise got to be too much. The kids weren't sleeping like they used to, which wasn't helping anyone. Brendan finally put his foot down. He was smart and insisted on some calm and an end to the chaos. Kelley could see he was right. They started to enforce some limitations on the well-meaning intrusions on their lives. It was time to start getting back to normal.

Breast cancer is a part of Kelley's family, and it will never go away. The kids see Kelley's stomach scar and mismatched breasts. They have asked about them, and Kelley says they are the scars from the operation where the doctor got rid of Mommy's cancer. She doesn't hide the breast cancer, nor does she bring it up every day. Ultimately, Kelley wants her kids to know how hard she fought to be alive for them and how much they inspired her every single day.

COUPLES

If you are married, your husband may feel like he comes at the bottom of your list at times. A serious illness can put a strain on a marriage. It forces you both to take a good look at your relationship. Your commitment will be tested as you find out if those vows really did mean something.

Marriages that were fragile to begin with can break. This is a very stressful time. If you haven't noticed, there isn't a lot out there focusing on the breast cancer husband. Cancer centers will tell you they don't have support groups for men because no one comes.

Kelley was worried about Brendan so she asked a survivor friend to have her husband call and talk with him. She just wanted to make sure his concerns were being heard. A lot of times Brendan felt like Kelley's family and friends were swooping in to the rescue, leaving him struggling to find his place.

But Kelley thought Brendan did a wonderful job of simply keeping everything together. She wanted him to keep working and doing well at his job. She wanted him to be there for the kids when she could not be there. Kelley knew she could find companionship or conversation elsewhere. It was reassuring to know Brendan was keeping everything running at home.

Brendan and Kelley tried to stay close and stay calm. They really focused on keeping organized and not letting anything with the kids fall through the cracks.

Try to nurture your marriage during this time of stress. When you feel well, make time for a date night and talk about anything other than cancer. Get away for a few hours or a few days and reconnect in a place that's as far away from a hospital setting as you can get.

Fighting cancer can be a long process and can require some major adjustments to your lifestyle. You will tolerate these changes because you will do anything to save your life. But remember it's not easy for your spouse or partner either. The disruptions in both of your lives can become hard to accept. Patience and communication become so important at this time. This is a new chapter in a couple's life and it will take time to adjust to it. Sometimes your spouse might feel shut out because, let's face it, only someone who has walked in our shoes really knows how it feels to fight this monster. Sometimes other survivors or other women in our lives simply take on a more prominent role. That's what we women do for one another.

ELISHA: When all my hair finally fell out, Doug went out and had his hair shaved off. At first I was furious! How could he shave off all those gorgeous blond curls? But then I realized what a sweet, generous gesture it was. In his own way, he was trying to share an experience with me.

I tried to keep life as normal as possible when I was feeling good. When I was having an off day, I just had to give into that, too. The most important thing is to do what you can when you can. Try not to punish yourself when you can't.

We've told you this before, but it is important to remember that this is the one time in your life to focus on yourself and your healing. But do try to keep your spouse or partner close. You need this person more than ever right now. And many couples emerge from this experience stronger than before. Your love and commitment to each other is an important part of getting through treatment.

CAREERS

We are both women who love what we do for a living. Our careers are part of who we are and how we believe we contribute to the world. We did not want to let cancer take away all that we had worked so hard to achieve.

When Kelley interviewed Robin Roberts of *Good Morning America* on WCVB-TV, she asked her why she kept working during treatment. "I get to be me from 7 until 9 a.m.," Robin said. "I'm myself again."

If that's how you feel, or if you need to work to pay your bills or get insurance coverage, we will share with you how we pulled it off. But we know every patient is different, and chemotherapy affects us all differently. If you struggle with fatigue, nausea, or low blood counts, work may not be an option. You have to do what's best for you, your family, and your health. Certain jobs may not be possible to do while undergoing treatment. Every situation is unique.

You might want to start by having a conversation with your boss. Try to be up-front about what you expect in terms of treatment. Then you will need to talk to him or her or someone in human resources about sick leave policies.

The Americans with Disabilities Act (ADA) is a federal law that applies to employers with fifteen or more employees. A person is protected by the ADA if she has a physical or mental impairment that substantially limits a major life function. To qualify, a person must be able to perform the essential functions of the job, with reasonable accommodation, if necessary (which must be provided by the employer as long as it does not create any undue hardship for the employer).

We asked Kathryn Joyce of the Disability Law Center Inc. some questions about your rights in the workplace.

Q: Are breast cancer patients protected under the Americans with Disabilities Act?

A: It depends. Under the ADA, there is no list of "automatic" disabilities. Rather, there is a definition of disability, which must be applied individually on a case-by-case basis. To qualify as a person with a disability under the ADA, an individual must:

- Have a physical or mental impairment that substantially limits one or more major life activities;
- Have a record of such an impairment; or
- Be regarded as having such an impairment.

Examples of major life activities are hearing, seeing, speaking, walking, breathing, performing manual tasks, sleeping, standing, caring for oneself, learning, concentrating, thinking, and working. In addition, major life activities include the proper functioning of major bodily functions, such as the immune and digestive systems, bowel, neurological, respiratory, circulatory, or endocrine functions, and normal cell growth.

A person with breast cancer would likely meet the ADA's definition of disability because her cancer substantially limits the major life activity of normal cell growth. In addition, a woman undergoing treatment for breast cancer may experience side effects of such treatment, including nausea or fatigue, that substantially limit her major life activities of caring for herself, sleeping, or concentrating.

Q: Do you have examples of reasonable accommodations a patient might expect from an employer during treatment?

A: Reasonable accommodations are changes, adjustments, or modifications to an employee's job or workspace, or to an employer's policies or practices, which allow an employee with a disability an equal opportunity to perform the essential functions of his or her job. An employer must provide accommodations that are needed because of a person's cancer or because of the side effects of medication or treatment for cancer.

Examples of employment accommodations that a woman may need as a result of having breast cancer are:

- Leave to recuperate from treatment;
- Flexible scheduling to attend doctors' appointments;
- A part-time schedule to manage cancer treatments;
- Periodic breaks to rest or take medication;
- Permission to work from home;
- Modification of office temperature or ventilation;
- Reassignment of marginal (nonessential) job tasks to other employees;
- Reassignment to another open position for which she is qualified; and/or
- Redesign of a workspace to be more ergonomically appropriate.

Q: **How should a patient inform an employer about a diagnosis and ask for accommodations?**

A: There are no "magic words" that an employee must use when requesting a workplace accommodation. An employee need only provide enough information to an employer to make it clear that she has a disability and needs a change or adjustment to her work or workspace. However, it is advisable that an employee who has a disability and needs a reasonable accommodation make her request in writing and include the following information:

- Identify the disability;
- State that reasonable accommodation(s) is/are being requested pursuant to the Americans with Disabilities Act;
- Identify the specific job tasks or workplace conditions affected by the disability;
- Provide one or more examples of accommodations that would reduce or eliminate the problem(s);
- Request that the employer discuss your accommodation ideas with you;
- Provide medical documentation to confirm the fact that you have a disability and to support your request for the specific accommodation(s) you have proposed; and
- Request that your employer respond in writing within a reasonable amount of time.

Some employers may have forms that can be used by an employee who needs reasonable accommodation. Otherwise, an informal letter to a supervisor, HR professional, or other individual with decision-making authority is appropriate.

An excellent resource for advice and ideas regarding workplace reasonable accommodation is the Job Accommodation Network (http://www.jan.wvu.edu).

Q: What should a patient do if she thinks her rights are being violated?

A: A person who believes that they have been discriminated against because of a disability may file a charge of discrimination with the U.S. Equal Employment Opportunity Commission. Also, most states have administrative agencies that investigate claims of employment discrimination. Short deadlines apply, so a person who thinks she may have been discriminated against should seek advice and consider filing a claim as soon thereafter as possible.

The Family and Medical Leave Act is a federal law that allows an employee to take up to twelve weeks of unpaid medical leave during any twelve-month period without losing her job or health insurance coverage. It applies to employers with fifty or more employees, and the employee must have worked at the company for at least one year. This leave can be tailored to the needs of your treatment.

You may qualify for long-term disability, which usually includes a reduction in pay, but you keep benefits.

Another option may be short-term disability. Every plan is different, but this is a period of paid leave typically based on years of service.

Kelley's employer allowed her to use short-term disability days as necessary. They were all in a "bank," so to speak, and Kelley used them as needed. She took four weeks off for surgery. During AC, she took off the chemo week and then worked the next two. During Taxol, she took off every Monday for treatment. Kelley was back to full-time work by the time radiation rolled around. But fatigue became a problem, and she scaled back to four days a week about halfway through.

Kelley based her work schedule on the advice of her doctor, survivors, and the goodwill of station management. It worked out very well. She knew she did not want to go on long-term disability. She wanted to work and she was particularly committed to allowing viewers to follow her progress during treatment both on TV and online. But she knew she needed time to recover from these punishing treatments. Kelley is grateful her employer allowed her to find a plan that worked for all involved.

It is your choice whether to disclose your medical condition to your employer. If you do not require some type of accommodation, you are not obligated to disclose your illness. Some employees are concerned that if they tell their employers they have cancer, they will be treated differently or will face discrimination.

Early in your diagnosis, you won't know how your body will react to a treatment until it happens. At a minimum, you will want to keep your options open. You may just want to keep lines of communication open with your employer. Don't put too much pressure on yourself. If a treatment is causing more side effects than you expected, speak up and take the time or other accommodations you need. Don't be a martyr at the expense of your recovery and healing.

ELISHA: To say that I am a workaholic is a complete understatement. My career has never simply been a job to me; it is my lifestyle. It has always come before anything else in my life. I'm not recommending this as a way of life for anyone, but it's how things were for me. One's life is made up of the decisions we make, and I chose my career over everything else. A cancer diagnosis quickly changed all that, but in the meantime I had to figure out how to juggle my busy career and my new part-time job, which was trying to save my life. I decided to figure out how to do both.

First you need to try to get your employer to understand the challenges you face. I was very lucky that my boss is a huge champion of women's causes. Sara Campbell was amazingly understanding of my new crazy schedule.

You will quickly learn when your body will need to recover from treatment and when you will be well enough for work. For instance, I had AC chemo every other Wednesday afternoon. I was fine on Thursday, but by Friday afternoon I was struggling. Saturday and Sunday I usually spent on the couch. By the following week, I would rally and get on with my life until the next treatment. The effects of chemo are cumulative, so it gets harder to rally back each time—but you will! Your body may have a different response that you will have to adjust to.

I also realized quickly that although fighting my cancer had to be my number one priority for now, it was only a moment in time and it would not be this way forever. No one is defined by any one thing in her life, and we should all get to live a few different chapters in our lives. I'm glad I kept working through treatment because I knew there had to be life before, during, and after cancer!

OTHER CHALLENGES

Cancer treatment will likely take a toll on you financially, even if you have insurance. Many hospital stays and treatments can come with deductibles and extra charges. Co-pays, transportation, parking, and child care can add up. Paying for prescription drugs can be a struggle. Wigs, as we have mentioned, are expensive.

If you find yourself struggling to stay on top of the bills, don't ignore the problem. It will not go away. You or someone you love must deal with the situation. Contact the mortgage company, credit card, or medical provider and explain what's going on.

If you are uninsured or underinsured, sit down with a social worker at your cancer center who can direct you to appropriate resources. You will also want to speak to someone in the hospital's billing department to see if they can assist you or work out a payment plan.

If you do not have a lot of support, contact one of the amazing organizations listed at the end of the book. There is help out there and you are not alone.

Don't Lose Your Sanity!

- Keep lines of communication open with your family, friends, and employer.
- Get help at the cancer center or at school if your children are not coping well with your treatment.
- Figure out what you need in terms of workplace accommodations and then ask your employer to work with you.
- Don't push yourself too hard. You have a lot going on and need to take care of yourself first.

Don't Lose Your Style!

- Work or keep up your regular routine when possible. It may help you feel like your old self again.
- Try to find some time to do activities that rejuvenate your body and spirit.
- Feel free to cut back on obligations that you don't want to take on right now. Instead of going to that boring meeting, take time out to go for a walk or a nap!
- Find ways to nurture your relationships with your family. Do simple activities that remind all of you that there is still a lot to celebrate in your life. Go to the beach, go for an easy hike, or watch a movie together on the couch.

ELEVEN

Sex and Fertility

Cancer treatment tends to take a lot of steam out of anyone's sex life. It starts with the shock of the diagnosis and goes downhill from there. It's tough to even think about sex when you have so much on your plate.

Let's start with the surgically altered body. It's certainly not easy for a woman or her partner to adjust to what may be big changes in physical appearance. You will probably have to learn to adjust to your new body first and then encourage your partner or potential partners to do the same. Any of us can admit these changes are not ideal, but the most important thing is to survive this disease. You can learn new ways of finding pleasure in an intimate relationship despite the physical changes you are enduring.

ELISHA: As hard as cancer treatment is on a patient, it can be just as difficult for a spouse, partner, or loved one to see you in such distress. I know Doug suffered a lot during my treatment as well. He had to focus on work while also picking up the slack on all the things I suddenly couldn't do. He got very little attention, and the last thing I wanted to do was have sex. I was certainly not feeling particularly fabulous. My bald head and my one boob were definitely throwing things off. I had to continuously remind myself that this was not all about me. It took me some time, but I finally realized that Doug's needs and desires didn't just disappear because I got breast cancer. He needed physical contact with me now more than ever. In the end, I felt so much more secure in our relationship and in our marriage after going through it with him and taking his needs into account sometimes.

Take It Slow

It takes time to regain your footing after being diagnosed with breast cancer. Don't rush into having sexual relations until you are ready. Take time to get comfortable with yourself and your new body. Also, make sure you feel well enough for sexual activity. If it has been a while, make time to get reacquainted with your partner. Go away together or find some time when you feel well, can relax, and can be left alone. Then take your time rediscovering sex.

Being sick can often make you feel so removed from life as you once knew it. Having sex with your partner is one way to celebrate being alive. You are doing something for pure enjoyment.

At first, you may find sex is not as enjoyable as it was precancer. You may feel self-conscious about your new body. Keep the lights dimmed if that makes you feel more comfortable. Find lingerie that works with your altered physique. And by all means keep communication lines open with your lover. Be straightforward about what feels good and bad, and share your feelings about your body.

Chemo can cause many women to stop getting their periods. Hormone therapies can also have side effects such as hot flashes and vaginal dryness. Yes, this is yet another wonderful gift from your breast cancer. You may find your plunging estrogen levels will send your libido south as well. Sex, which was once fun, may become more of a chore.

Sanity Saver

Think about what makes you feel sexy. Is it something you wear? Is it somewhere you go? Dancing? Can you go back to a place that was once the setting for a steamy night? Can you rent a sexy movie? With a little effort you may be able to jump-start your libido.

HOT FLASHES

If your hot flashes are intense, have a talk with your oncologist. He or she may be able to prescribe low-dose antidepressants or other medications to lessen the hot flashes. It probably goes without saying that your breast cancer means you may not be a candidate for the hormone replacement therapies that some other women use to combat the effects of menopause. But we both know firsthand that hot flashes can be a major disruption to your life—especially to your sleep. Speak up if you are steaming up. Don't suffer silently.

HIGH AND DRY

If vaginal dryness is a problem you will definitely want to talk with your oncologist or gynecologist. There is no need to suffer through sex. That is just not fun. Dr. Partridge recommends her patients try a water-based lubricant such as Replens. This estrogen-free product is more like a moisturizer and lasts up to three days. You may also want to experiment with other lubricants to see what works best. This is one way to turn a negative into something that might bring a little spice back to your bedroom.

Play It Safe

Even if your periods are irregular or have stopped, you may still be fertile. To be safe, you should talk to your doctor about a hormone-free birth control method. You don't need the stress of an unplanned pregnancy on top of everything else that's going on right now.

Fertility

For premenopausal women a breast cancer diagnosis can bring another level of pain. You may not have had a chance to start your family yet or may not be done having children. Obviously every cancer case is different, and you should speak to your oncologist about fertility issues. Dr. Partridge, who founded and directs the Program for Young Women with Breast Cancer at Dana-Farber, focuses her research and care on the unique issues facing this group. Here is some of the advice she gives her patients about fertility.

Fertility and pregnancy are important concerns for many young women with breast cancer. Chemotherapy and other treatments may affect ovarian function, menstrual periods, and fertility. These treatments' effects are outlined briefly below, as well as various approaches to preserving fertility. If you think you might want to become pregnant in the future, talk to your physician about the risks of infertility associated with various treatments and the options for trying to preserve your fertility.

One possible side effect of breast cancer treatment is amenorrhea (not having periods), which may result in loss of fertility. The risk of amenorrhea from chemotherapy depends on a woman's age and the specific drug regimen used. It is important to understand that amenorrhea may be temporary, lasting for a number of months, or permanent, resulting in menopause.

For most women, if periods have not resumed within the first year after treatment, amenorrhea is permanent. Women whose periods continue after chemotherapy may go through menopause earlier than they would have if they had not received the treatment. However, the presence or absence of periods during the first several months after chemotherapy is not the best indicator of fertility. The return of menstrual cycles does not necessarily mean that the ovaries are producing normal eggs that will result in a healthy pregnancy, and the absence of menstrual cycles after chemotherapy does not necessarily mean that fertility has been permanently lost. You should speak to your physician if you are concerned about whether you can become pregnant after chemotherapy. There are some factors that may help determine if you will be fertile posttreatment.

- Effect of age: Fertility declines naturally as a woman ages. Women over the age of forty are more likely than younger women to have amenorrhea as a result of chemotherapy, and amenorrhea is more likely to be permanent in older women.
- Effect of drug regimen: Common chemotherapy regimens for breast cancer can have various effects on the risk of amenorrhea, early menopause, and resulting loss of fertility. These effects are also related to age, as noted above.

If you have questions about the likelihood of going through menopause with your treatment, you should consult your physician and consider this risk in making decisions about treatment.

Please note that pregnancy can occur during treatment with chemotherapy and tamoxifen but is not safe because of an increased risk of birth defects and miscarriage, particularly in the first trimester. Therefore, effective barrier contraception is strongly recommended during chemotherapy.

Tamoxifen is a hormonal therapy that is often used in women with estrogen receptor–positive breast cancer. Treatment with tamoxifen is usually given over a period of several years to block the action of estrogen and potentially stop or slow the growth of cancer cells. Tamoxifen treatment generally does not cause early menopause; however, periods can become irregular. Furthermore, because the use of tamoxifen and other endocrine therapies is often recommended for several years, fertility may naturally decline with age during this time.

Suppressing (shutting down) the ovaries can help prevent breast cancer from coming back in premenopausal women with hormone receptor–positive breast cancer. There are three ways to suppress the ovaries: surgery, radiation, and injections of drugs known as LHRH (luteinizing hormone–releasing hormone) analogues, such as leuprolide, goserelin, and triptorelin. If drug injections are used to suppress ovarian function, they are usually given for a number of years.

Surgery and radiation shut down the ovaries permanently, resulting in loss of fertility. If LHRH analogues are used for ovarian suppression, it is likely that the ovaries will start working again once the injections are stopped. The most common side effects of these drugs are hot flashes, amenorrhea, decreased sex drive, vaginal dryness, painful intercourse, and bone thinning.

LHRH analogues can affect an unborn baby; therefore, such drugs must not be used in pregnant women, and effective barrier contraception is strongly recommended. These drugs should also not be used in women who are breast-feeding.

Preserving Your Fertility

It is difficult to know whether you will be fertile after undergoing treatment for breast cancer. However, there are steps that you can take before treatment that may help preserve your fertility. If you think you might want to become pregnant, ask your physician which of these options would be best for you and when it would be safe to become pregnant. You may also want to consider an early referral to a reproductive endocrinologist (fertility specialist), who can help you further understand your fertility choices. It is important to note that the choices are imperfect; options don't always work and may be quite difficult.

Options include:

- Freezing embryos (requires sperm)
- Freezing eggs or a piece of ovary (very experimental)
- Taking ovarian suppresion shots (experimental, not clear if it works)

For more information, go to the Fertile Hope Website (http://www.fertile hope.org).

Pregnancy after Breast Cancer

Women of childbearing age diagnosed with breast cancer, along with their many treatment concerns, now have the unique concern related to fertility and family planning. Today, there are many options available, and talking with your oncologist about these issues can be very helpful with this important decision.

Although research in this area is limited, research studies have not shown an increased risk of cancer returning in women who have had a pregnancy after breast cancer compared to those who have not. Furthermore, children born after treatment for breast cancer seem to have no increased risk of birth defects.

Many oncologists encourage patients to delay childbearing between two to five years after the completion of the first treatment for breast cancer. This is because the majority of young women who develop recurrent breast cancer do so within the first five years of diagnosis, with the most aggressive cancers recurring within the first two to three years. Further, most young women with hormone receptor-positive breast cancer will be advised to take hormonal therapy for several years, during which time they should not become pregnant.

BREAST-FEEDING

The ability to breast-feed after treatment for breast cancer depends on the individual and on the treatment received. Women who have been treated for breast cancer and deliver a child can usually breast-feed.

Most women who have undergone radiation treatment are able to produce milk on the affected breast; however, the milk production may not be adequate enough, and breast-feeding may be limited to the untreated breast.

Breast-feeding during active treatment with chemotherapy or tamoxifen is not recommended. Many anticancer drugs, such as cyclophosphamide and methotrexate, may occur in high levels in breast milk and may harm the nursing baby.

Getting a referral to a reproductive endocrinologist is important if you are interested in having a biological child after breast cancer diagnosis and treatment, and are having difficulty getting pregnant after treatment.

ELISHA: I can't be the only woman who thought I had all the time in the world to have a child. Then, suddenly, I was diagnosed with breast cancer, and my life changed forever. Doug and I got married young by today's standards. I was twenty-two years old and he was twenty-four. We traveled around the world. We built our careers and moved around. Basically, we have always been busy living a full life. I always assumed that when it was meant to be we would have a baby. We always thought we had plenty of time.

Suddenly I was forty years old and diagnosed with breast cancer. Knowing I no longer had any control over whether we had a baby was so much more devastating to me than I ever expected. I had to face the fact that an opportunity in my life had passed me by, and I would have to live with that forever. I learned to focus on the fact that I did have a second opportunity to live a healthy, full life with the man I love.

We learn to cope with the limitations our cancer brings to our lives while celebrating the victories big and small. Kelley had just given birth to her second child and would find out she would not be able to have any more. Her five years of tamoxifen would put her at age forty-two and likely past her childbearing years. Kelley also opted for a TRAM reconstruction, and pregnancy after such surgery is not recommended.

KELLEY: Brendan and I were on the fence about having a third child. We both worked and felt two may be all we could handle. However, it was upsetting to have cancer take away the possibility of more children. It was one more layer to this crisis that was difficult to swallow. Doctors pointed out that we could adopt another child if we wanted to. For a while, I would find myself on adoption Web sites looking at children. Then I came to realize I had enough on my plate without taking on an adoption project. I spent some time being angry that cancer had made this crucial life decision for me. With time I learned to be very grateful that my second daughter, Cecilia, was born before we found the lump. If not, we wouldn't have this amazing child in our lives. These personal feelings take a while to process. Give yourself time to sort it all out.

Adoption is always an option to consider once you have finished treatment if a biological child is not a reasonable option for you. Allow yourself to heal and then begin considering your options. You still have the ability to make your dreams of having a family come true. It just may not be exactly how you envisioned it.

Don't Lose Your Sanity!

- When it comes to sex, take it slow. Your body may feel different, so take your time.
- Find the right time to resume your sex life. Plan a night away or simply find some downtime where you can feel relaxed.
- You don't have to love your new body; you just have to learn to accept it.
- Remember that partners have needs, too, and communicate, communicate, communicate!
- If you think you might be interested in having a baby after breast cancer, speak to your doctor before you are treated about the risks of treatment to your fertility. Consider early referral to a fertility specialist and fertility preservation techniques if warranted.

Don't Lose Your Style!

- Treat yourself to some fabulous new lingerie. Anything that makes you feel pretty right now.
- Put a little more effort into romance—scented candles or flowers in your bedroom.
- On one of your "good" nights, plan a romantic evening out with your husband or partner.

TWELVE

Hormone Therapy and Moving On

If you're like us, you may have struggled at times with the word "survivor." Technically you're supposed to call yourself a survivor the minute you are diagnosed. Kelley jokes that you should be called a survivor if you didn't have a heart attack when they said you had cancer!

Now that you have gone through surgery, maybe chemo, and perhaps radiation, you are definitely a survivor. You now join more than ten million Americans living with a history of cancer. Emphasis, of course, on living.

Sometimes a terrible experience such as breast cancer inspires you to do something new and wonderful. If you can survive this, you can survive anything. As horrific as breast cancer is to endure, it may ultimately change who you are for the better. We learned a lot through our cancer experiences, but one of the main lessons was to no longer have any fear. There is something amazingly liberating about knowing you have faced and conquered the most terrifying challenge of your life.

Hormone Therapy

In order to improve your chances of living a long, cancer-free life your oncologist may prescribe hormone therapy. That's because the female hormones estrogen and progesterone can promote the growth of some breast cancer cells. Hormone therapy is given to block or lower the body's naturally occurring estrogen and fight the cancer's growth. For women with hormone receptor-positive breast cancer, hormone therapy often reduces the risk of recurrence more than chemotherapy. Hormone therapy is not appropriate, however, for someone diagnosed with hormone receptor–negative cancer. Keep in mind that hormone therapy is not to be confused with hormone replacement therapy. Hormone therapy for cancer treatment stops hormones from getting to cancer cells. Hormone replacement therapy for postmenopausal women without cancer adds more hormones to your body to counter the effects of menopause.

There are three types of hormone therapy for breast cancer. Tamoxifen and other drugs like it block estrogen and progesterone from promoting breast cancer cell growth. Aromatase inhibitors, including Arimidex (anastrozole), Femara (letrozole), and Aromasin (exemestane), decrease the production of estrogen in postmenopausal women. And LHRH-agonist drugs, including Zoladex (goserelin), Lupron (leuprolide), and Trelstar (triptorelin), as well as surgery or radiation, can be used to suppress ovarian production of estrogens in a premenopausal woman.

Tamoxifen

Tamoxifen is a once-a-day pill that decreases the chance that hormone receptor–positive, early stage breast cancers will recur by slowing or stopping the growth of cancer cells that may be present in the body. It can prevent the development of a new cancer in the unaffected breast.

Tamoxifen is a type of drug called a selective estrogen receptor modulator (SERM). At the breast, it functions as an anti-estrogen agent. Estrogen promotes the growth of breast cancer cells, and tamoxifen blocks estrogen from attaching to estrogen receptors on these cells. It is believed that this halts the growth of the breast cancer cells.

SIDE EFFECTS

The side effects of tamoxifen may be similar to the symptoms of menopause. The most common complaints women have are hot flashes and vaginal discharge. Other side effects may include irregular menstrual periods, headaches, nausea, skin rashes, fatigue, and the dreaded weight gain.

Many women complain about weight gain on tamoxifen. Dr. Partridge will tell you that research has revealed that women are just as likely to gain weight on tamoxifen as they are on a placebo (a sugar pill!). But she believes every patient when they tell her that their tamoxifen is making them gain weight or preventing them from losing the pounds they may have put on during chemotherapy (research here shows that the chemo actually does cause weight gain). She is adamant, however, that the therapy is too important for most women to give up merely to shrink your waistline. We're talking about your life, ladies! You will get the usual advice to exercise and eat a healthy diet, and for most women who actually do it, it usually works, at least to a degree.

RISKS

Tamoxifen may affect your periods, but you may still be fertile. You may want to use a barrier-type of birth control while on this medication. Women taking tamoxifen may have a slightly increased risk of developing blood clots in the lungs or large veins. There's also an increased risk of stroke, uterine cancer, and cataracts.

Dr. Partridge says the risks of a major problem are small and need to be balanced against the benefits of taking this lifesaving drug.

OTHER HORMONE THERAPIES

Aromatase inhibitors block the effect of an enzyme that helps the body produce estrogen. Aromatase inhibitors delay the progression of breast cancer to a greater degree than tamoxifen in postmenopausal women with advanced breast cancer whose tumors rely on estrogen to grow. In women with early stage, hormone receptor–positive disease, aromatase inhibitors may be used as part of the initial or follow-up treatment. They are pills that are taken once a day.

Side effects can include menopausal symptoms such as hot flashes and vaginal dryness, bone thinning, aches in your muscles and joints, nausea, weight gain, and headaches.

LHRH agonists stop the production of estrogen from the ovaries in premenopausal women. They are used for the treatment of women with estrogen-sensitive breast cancer. Side effects include menopausal symptoms such as hot flashes, vaginal dryness, bone thinning, and temporary cessation of periods.

Your oncologist will discuss the most appropriate options for you and come up with a treatment plan. It's vital that you follow the plan for the recommended time period, usually five years. For most women with hormone receptor–positive breast cancer, hormone treatment is one of the most important, greatest risk-reducing options. Find a time of day that you will always remember to take your pill. Keep the bottle by the coffee maker or your toothbrush so you won't forget.

Transitioning Out of Treatment

You probably think the end of treatment should be one big, happy celebration. But you may actually feel depressed. It's not easy to go from having lots of treatment to feeling like you are flying without a net. Treatment, as strange as it may sound, provides comfort because you know you are fighting the cancer. Now you're just waiting and praying the treatment worked.

Moving on can be the most joyous, exciting time and the most terrifying time all at once! You have to transition from being a cancer patient who is being treated and taken care of to being a survivor and on your own. Worrying constantly "Am I really cured?" can cripple you. You cannot play those mind games. Instead, focus on all the positive things in your life. This can be an opportunity to start your life all over again. Be grateful for it.

KELLEY: I was so spent by the time treatment was over. Brendan said we limped across the finish line. The exhaustion was taxing both physically and mentally. I thought I would rejuvenate myself by going away to the Berkshire Mountains in western Massachusetts for a yoga retreat. I spent a lot of that weekend crying. I would go for a walk in the woods and just cry. I mean sobbing, uncontrollable tears. It was horrible. I wondered if there would ever come a day when I didn't worry about my cancer coming back. I didn't know if I would ever stop worrying about abandoning my two young children and husband. Each day did get a bit easier, and the fear started to subside. It just took a while to get the old Kelley back.

Rebuilding Your Life

You have to come to terms with all that has happened and how your life has changed. Once you can really process your cancer experience, you can move forward. Cancer causes you to look at life a bit differently. You may want to take stock of your relationships and your job and how you spend your time, or you may just want to resume where you left off.

There are some steps you should probably take in order to improve your chances of putting all this behind you once and for all. Exercising, losing weight if overweight, and improving your diet are always good goals for optimal health. Nevertheless, doctors caution that so far the research on lifestyle and dietary changes after breast cancer have not yet been definitively proven to improve outcomes.

Exercise

Exercise definitely should be a part of a healthy postcancer lifestyle. One 2005 study showed that walking three to five hours a week at a pace of two to three miles per hour during and after treatment was associated with a lower risk for recurrence and death by up to 40 percent. Neither one of us liked to exercise before, but, trust us, we make time now. It's too important to blow off. If you are wiped out from treatment, start slowly. Take a walk in your neighborhood and gradually increase the duration and frequency as you get stronger. Buy some weights or join a gym. Resistance exercise is very important for those of us who have been treated for cancer. You have to protect and strengthen your bones. Some YMCAs now offer the Pink Program, a twelve-week fitness plan designed especially for survivors designed by our friend and survivor Dr. Carolyn Kaelin.

Elisha started a regime of power walking three miles a day, five days a week, shortly after treatment. It's now a part of her daily routine.

Be patient with yourself posttreatment. Kelley can remember going swimming with her young daughter at the town pond. She started heading toward the dock and quickly realized with fear that she wasn't sure she had the strength or stamina to make it. It was a frightening and humbling experience.

Kelley's friend A. T. Palmer is a survivor living in Chicago. She wrote a wonderful e-mail about getting back to the gym three years after being diagnosed with breast cancer.

Sat around this morning stewing at home, inventing work, afraid to go over, knew I had to. Finally, around noon, realized it couldn't be postponed any more. Threw the stuff in a gym bag and headed over. Meandered down to the gals' locker room where I had to make my first decision. Was I going into a dressing room or dressing out in the open, the way I used to? Used to won out. If there's a woman in the locker room who'd been delaying her mammogram, looking at me all stitched up (with my nipple tattoo!), maybe that would motivate her.

Gravitated to the treadmill first, an old friend. 4.5 mph, 4 percent incline, 15 minutes for a start, enough to work up a sweat. First one in three years! Boy, did it feel good to smell crummy again!

Then I played with some of the machines for another half hour— hip abductor, adductor, upper body strengthening. Until I needed a treat—steam bath!

That's when I couldn't stop crying. Don't know whether it was that I finally made it back there after so long, whether I realized how much I'd missed working out and really was strong enough to do this again, or whether it was because I'd gotten through the first day! But I'm definitely going back tomorrow.

NUTRITION

Hillary Wright, MEd, RD, LDN, a nutritionist at Dana-Farber Cancer Institute, says maintaining a healthy weight is associated with a significant reduction in risk of cancer recurrence. Studies show moderate weight loss in women who are overweight, 5 to 10 percent, may reduce risk. Body mass index (BMI) is one way to determine a healthy weight. The Centers for Disease Control has a BMI calculator at http://www.cdc.gov/nccdphp/dnpa/bmi/calc-bmi.htm. Wright says survivors should aim for a BMI of 20 to 25.

One of the best things you can do after treatment is to start or continue eating a healthy diet. Start by aiming for five or more servings of vegetables and fruits each day. Leave your sweet tooth behind, and pick up whole grain foods instead of white flour and sugars. Try to limit meats that are high in fat. Cut back on processed foods. Continue to drink plenty of water each day to stay adequately hydrated. The combination of healthy eating and exercise should help you maintain a weight that's appropriate for your body. Seek help from a cancer center nutritionist if you need it.

Wright says there is no scientific data linking growth hormone use in food production and cancer. But she has many patients who choose to buy organic foods. If cost is a concern, Wright suggests buying organic only for those foods believed to be most potentially contaminated. The Environmental Working Group, a consumer advocacy group, has produced a list of the most and least pesticide- and residue-contaminated fruits and vegetables, called the "Dirty Dozen" and the "Clean Fifteen," as a guide to help consumers know where to best spend their organic dollars. Check it out online at http://www.foodnews.org/walletguide.php.

Wright suggests you take a look at the fats in your diet. Try to include healthy fats like fish (salmon, flounder, herring, and sardines), olive and canola oils, nuts and nut butters, flax seed, wheat germ, and avocados.

And try to reduce "unfriendly" fats like whole milk products, butter and margarine, French fries and other deep-fried foods, pastries, crackers, and processed foods.

Many of you may be wondering if you can still eat soy after a breast cancer diagnosis. Wrights says isoflavones found in soy foods exert a weak, estrogen-like effect on the body. It's unknown if excessive consumption could fuel the growth of estrogen-positive cancer cells. She suggests survivors might want to avoid soy isofavone supplements, but whole soy foods (such as soymilk and tofu) can be eaten in moderation several times a week.

ELISHA: We've already told you that cancer will change you forever, but how do you change yourself forever? If you are a control freak like me, you want to do anything you can to protect your body and your mind. It is very important to maintain a healthy weight. For much of my life, I suffered from an eating disorder. I thought this was my biggest problem until I was diagnosed with breast cancer. Suddenly I was fighting for my life in a different way. When I was diagnosed with breast cancer, I weighed about ninety-four pounds, which on a five-foot-six frame was completely unhealthy. It suddenly became so important to me to eat healthy and to exercise regularly, two things I had never done before. During my chemo treatment I started walking every day. Every morning that I had enough energy to walk, I did. And I always felt better after it. Exercise also helped me maintain a healthy weight after chemo treatment pushed me into early menopause and tamoxifen packed on the pounds.

Vitamin D

Though not definitive, some studies found that women with adequate vitamin D levels have lower rates of breast cancer. Check with your doctor to see if you are getting enough vitamin D. A simple blood test can check your levels. Dr. Partridge recommends her patients get between four hundred and eight hundred international units per day, based on the current research.

You absorb vitamin D through exposure to sunlight, but many of us wear sunscreen. It's tough to get all your vitamin D through food because sources are limited. Vitamin D is in fortified foods such as milk and cereals. Fatty fish is another source. You will probably want to consider supplements to ensure you are getting enough each day.

Alcohol

Watch what you drink. Studies show even moderate amounts of alcohol can increase your risk of breast cancer. You will probably want to take a look at how much alcohol you consume each week and consider substituting some sparkling water for some of that wine, bubbles, or beer! Generally, no more than one drink per day on average is recommended.

Stress

Stress is simply not healthy. Moving forward from cancer treatment may be a good time to look at the stress in your life and how you might reduce it. Those wellness techniques that may have helped you through treatment will continue to serve you as you move on. Can you make time in your schedule for yoga? There are spas and massage therapists everywhere in a variety of price ranges. Acupuncture has many amazing benefits; so does Reiki. If money is an issue, teach yourself how to meditate. These will all be good tools to have as you transition from patient to survivor.

Dealing with the Fear

With each cold, ache, or pain, you may find the fear that the cancer has returned creeping in. It's hard not to overreact to a simple ailment now that you have been touched by cancer. One survivor says she notes any pain or problem and refuses to worry about it for at least a week. If the problem is particularly severe, unusual, persists, or is getting worse over time, then you can contact a doctor. The fears do diminish over time. You just have to be patient with yourself. We all have to learn to live with some amount of uncertainty. You can control only certain things, but breast cancer, as we all know, may be ultimately out of your control.

Scans

Some of us would love to never have another scan in our lives. Others want the reassurance of a clean bill of health. Again, it's a strange feeling to finish treatment and assume you are cancer free but have no proof. Dr. Partridge does not routinely scan her patients after treatment. Randomized studies have shown that routine scanning and blood work in patients who are asymptomatic does not improve long-term outcomes or quality of life. Most people who develop recurrent disease (75 percent) in those studies actually presented with symptoms between scans and blood work in the group that was getting scanned. So even with intensive scanning, you are more likely than not to miss the cancer before it has become symptomatic. And, on average, in those studies, disease was only picked up a month earlier in the patients whose cancer returned in the screened group versus the unscreened group. So without a change in overall survival, with all of the above issues, Dr. Partridge recommends against scanning for asymptomatic people because it has the potential to generate not only anxiety, but a false sense of security (my scans were fine last month so this worsening back pain couldn't be disease—I am not going to call the doc), as well as nuisance, possible additional unnecessary testing including biopsies, and exorbitant health care costs.

Dr. Partridge's bottom line: Unfortunately, early detection of distant recurrent breast cancer does not improve outcomes. If cancer is going to come back elsewhere in the body, picking it up with a symptom versus an asymptomatic scan will not change in general how a person does in the long run. If treatment works, which it often does, then it will work when disease is detected either way, even if there is a little more disease in the person not being screened.

That being said, Dr. Partridge counsels patients not to bury their heads in the sand, and early attention to symptoms that are worsening over time or particularly strange or severe is prudent to prevent pain and suffering. But she points out that studies show the vast majority of symptoms in survivors that prompt scans are not associated with a recurrence.

Dr. Partridge sees patients every three to six months until they are no longer on therapy or reach the five-year mark. That is a milestone that many cancer patients view as an important one, though, unfortunately, some will experience a recurrence of their cancer after five years.

Standard follow-up guidelines have been assembled by an expert panel of the American Society of Clinical Oncologists (ASCO). A patient version of the guidelines is available at http://www.cancer.net.

Eventually, you will no longer need to see your oncologists regularly, but they are generally available to you on an as-needed basis. Let's hope you don't need them! You will continue your long-term survivorship care with your primary care doctor and/or gynecologist or other providers.

Protect Yourself Emotionally

Inevitably something will come up on the news or among your friends that will spark fear. You may hear about a public figure who has died of breast cancer. You may have a friend in a support group who has a recurrence. This isn't you or your cancer story, and you need to start protecting yourself so you can move forward. Have a strategy to change the conversation if someone approaches you with a story that makes you uncomfortable. Kelley had to stop reading obituaries in the newspaper because if she saw a breast cancer death, her mind would start reeling. She would want to know what exactly the woman had and how it was treated. If you find yourself dwelling on someone's cancer death, pick up Lance Armstrong's book *It's Not About the Bike* for inspiration. Learn to focus on all the incredible people living and thriving postcancer. You did not survive this disease to worry every day it will come back. Too much worrying can have a negative effect on the quality of your life.

Cancer recurrence is a possibility we all need to learn to live with. Kelley tells herself that even if the cancer returns, she has met many women living ten, fifteen, twenty years with metastatic disease. There are new treatments being discovered every day. Have hope that cancer will not return and have faith that you can handle any challenge you might face in the future. If fears get to be too much to handle, consider seeking professional help.

RELATIONSHIPS

Take stock of the loving support you received and try not to dwell on the people who disappointed you during your journey. Focus on the people who had your back and held you up. You will never forget how they inspired you to survive. Get back to work or your usual routine and be grateful for the return to normalcy. Remember that your body can still provide you with pleasure. We know that you've been through hell and back but you still have a ton of living to do. Some women may have difficulty with sex and intimate relationships after cancer treatment, but this will not last forever. It's okay to ask for professional help if you need it.

Gimme a Break!

Take a vacation—you deserve it! It is so important to reward yourself after all that you've been through. During your cancer treatment, you focus so much on getting through this time with your sanity in place. Give yourself some space to reflect on what has happened to you and celebrate how you have risen to the occasion with grace and style.

Sanity Saver

Many cancer centers and community programs offer postcancer workshops. They are designed to help women make the transition from patient to survivor. You may also connect with some other women who have just completed treatment and understand your fears and concerns. There are also great adventure programs geared toward women with breast cancer that we've listed at the end of the book. You definitely deserve a fly-fishing escape right about now!

Unexpected Gifts

Elisha still loves the latest Louis Vuitton bag or the hottest Jimmy Choo shoes. But she now treasures the confidence that comes from knowing you can survive and shine through a life-changing experience.

You may have been pleasantly surprised by the love and caring of family and friends. Your marriage or other relationships may be strengthened by the bond of going through such a trauma together. You may have new friends as a result of your illness. You likely share a bond and have deep gratitude for the doctors, nurses, and others who guided you through treatment. You have a renewed sense of self that comes from conquering a challenge that tested you unlike any other. It's hard not to be a better person for having survived breast cancer.

We told you: You can do this! And now you have. It's time to celebrate your strength, your courage, and your grace. Congratulations. We wish you a long, happy life.

Don't Lose Your Sanity!

- Remember, it will get easier with each passing day to get past the fears of the cancer returning. If it is not getting easier, speak to your doctors, who can refer you for counseling. Professional help may be your best option.
- Find a balance between having cancer be a part of your life through volunteer work and allowing yourself to move on.
- Continue to follow your doctors' instructions and take good care of yourself.
- Keep doing massage, exercise, and yoga to foster wellness in your postcancer life.

Don't Lose Your Style!

- Send a message to the world that you are back and better than ever!
- Resume your old life with a new purpose.
- Give back if you can. Remember somebody somewhere helped save your life.
- Inspire and mentor another woman to get through treatment with sanity and style. Just like you!

GENERAL AND MEDICAL INFORMATION

http://www.breastcancer.org
Wonderful Web site that's updated frequently and covers a wide variety of topics.

http://www.cancer.org
American Cancer Society's Web site, which includes a lot of information and resources available nationwide.

http://www.thebostonchannel.com/kelleys-story
Kelley Tuthill's video diary and blog. Also contains a lot of links to other breast cancer Web sites.

http://www.lbbc.org
Living Beyond Breast Cancer.

http://www.breastfree.org
For information about reconstruction or choosing to live without reconstruction.

http://www.mbcnetwork.org
Metastatic Breast Cancer Network.

http://www.tnbcfoundation.org
A Web site dedicated to those with triple negative breast cancer.

http://www.facingourrisk.org
A Web site for those with hereditary breast cancer.

http://www.ibcresearch.org
Inflammatory Breast Cancer Research Foundation.

http://www.youngsurvival.org
Young Survival Coalition Web site, which has information and resources geared toward those under forty.

http://www.cancer.net
American Society of Clinical Oncology.

http://www.cancer.gov
National Cancer Institute.

http://www.dana-farber.org
Dana-Farber Cancer Institute.

http://www.dana-farber.org/pat/adult/breast-cancer/program-for-young-women-with-breast-cancer
The Program for Young Women with Breast Cancer at Dana-Farber/Brigham and Women's Cancer Center.

http://www.fertilehope.org
Information about preserving fertility.

http://www.searchclinicaltrials.org
A clinical trials search portal.

http://www.clinicaltrials.gov
A registry of government and industry-sponsored clinical trials conducted in the United States and around the world.

http://www.centerwatch.com
Contains a large number of listings of industry-funded trials.

http://www.emergingmed.com
Clinical trials matching and referral service for cancer patients.

http://www.apta.org
American Physical Therapy Association.

Help Find a Cure

http://www.bcrfcure.org
The Breast Cancer Research Foundation.

http://www.stopbreastcancer.org
National Breast Cancer Coalition.

http://www.komen.org
Susan G. Komen for the Cure.

http://www.armyofwomen.org
Dr. Susan Love's Army of Women recruits women for studies across the country.

http://www.friendsofmel.org
The Friends of Mel Foundation has raised millions for breast cancer research and care by selling beautiful bracelets.

Help with Kids

http://www.cancer.org

American Cancer Society.

http://www.campkesem.org

A college-student-run summer camp for kids whose parents have cancer.

http://www.mghpact.org

Massachusetts General Hospital's Parenting at a Challenging Time program.

Surviving with Style

http://www.lookgoodfeelbetter.org

National program for women undergoing treatment.

http://www.hatandhair.com

Hats with detachable hair pieces.

http://lymphedivas.com

Fashionable compression sleeves.

http://www.healingthreads.com

Fashionable alternatives to the hospital johnny.

http://www.dearjohnnies.com

More cute alternatives to the hospital johnny.

http://www.headcovers.com

Head covers, makeup, and more.

http://www.saracampbell.com

Great pink clothes and fun items to benefit breast cancer research.

http://www.chikaradesign.com
Clothing for women experiencing breast asymmetry.

http://www.bra-cketbook.com
The Bra-cketbook Foundation has purses designed by a breast cancer survivor.

FINANCIAL ASSISTANCE

http://www.abcf.org
American Breast Cancer Foundation.

http://www.cancercare.org
Support for people with cancer.

http://www.healthwellfoundation.org
Helps patients afford treatment.

http://www.mowaa.org
Meals on Wheels.

http://www.myhopechest.org
Helps fund reconstructive surgery.

http://www.cancer.org
American Cancer Society.

http://www.rxassist.org
Provides free medications for those who cannot afford them.

http://www.cancerandcareers.org
A resource for working women with cancer.

GIVE ME A BREAK

http://www.castforthecure.org
Fly-fishing retreats for survivors.

http://www.firstdescents.org
Outdoor adventures for young survivors.

http://www.makingmemories.org
Grants wishes for metastatic patients.

http://www.stowehope.com
Weekend retreat in Vermont for survivors and families.

http://www.womenbeyondcancer.org
Retreats for survivors.

http://www.bjbbreastcancerretreats.org
Adventure-based retreats.

http://www.campdream.org
Offers a women's cancer retreat.

http://www.seasit.org
A nonprofit organization that promotes recovery through recreation for cancer patients who seek to recapture positive thinking and to regain control over their lives.

ACKNOWLEDGMENTS

Elisha and Kelley are deeply grateful for the participation of our oncologist, Dr. Ann Partridge. She not only took wonderful care of us during treatment but also recognized that this book was an important part of our healing and recovery. We are grateful for her time and expertise.

Thank you to Evelyn H. Lauder for her beautiful foreword and amazing work to solve the mysteries of this disease.

Our families made a lot of sacrifices so we could work on this project. Special thanks to our amazing husbands, Doug and Brendan, who know to stay out of the way when we set our minds to do something. We love them and thank them for their support. We also appreciate the support of our parents and extended family. Kelley's children, Madeline and Cecilia, drive all the work we do to make sure breast cancer is eliminated by the time they become adults.

We are grateful to all our caregivers who compassionately guided us through treatment. Many of them contributed to this book and we thank them.

Our medical and survival experts include Martie Carnie, Dr. Stephanie Caterson, Mary Flaherty, Kenneth Getz, Dr. Tim Moynihan, A. T. Palmer, Dr. Paula Rauch, Nancy Roberge, Dr. Julia Wong, and Hillary Wright. Rick DiCecca provided appearance advice, as did Nikki Walsh. Kathryn

Joyce and the Disability Law Center Inc. provided workplace information. Joel Benjamin was kind enough to take the beautiful photo on the back cover.

Our workplaces were good enough to support this project, and a big thank-you goes to our bosses and coworkers at Sara Campbell LTD and WCVB-TV Boston. Stephanie Millon and Erin Duggan were particularly helpful. We also thank our literary agent, Doe Coover.

Several friends and relatives gave us great advice on this project, including Nichole Bernier Ahern, Megan Colarossi, Kelley Doyle, Dr. Carolyn Kaelin, Dr. Julie Silver, and Andi Silverman.

The hero of this project is our editor, Christine Schillig, vice president and editorial director of the book division at Andrews McMeel Publishing. She recognized the potential of this book and agreed to take on two unpublished authors. Her vision, patience, and guidance made this project possible. We are forever grateful to her and all our friends at Andrews McMeel Publishing, especially John McMeel and Hugh Andrews.

This book is dedicated to Elisha's dear sister-in-law Marilyn Montiero. Her strength and bravery in fighting her own cancer was an inspiration to all who knew her. She will be forever in our hearts.